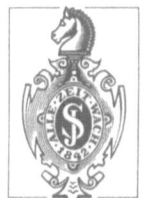

Treatment in Clinical Medicine
Series Editor: John L. Reid

Colin Feek · Christopher Edwards

Endocrine and Metabolic Disease

With 43 Figures

Springer-Verlag
London Berlin Heidelberg New York
Paris Tokyo

Colin M. Feek, MBBS, MRCP
Specialist Physician in Endocrinology, Wellington Hospital, Wellington 2,
New Zealand

Christopher R. W. Edwards, MD, FRCP, FRCP (Ed)
Professor of Clinical Medicine, University of Edinburgh Department of Medicine,
Western General Hospital, Edinburgh, Scotland

With a contribution by:
Allan D. Struthers, MBchB, MRCP
Senior Lecturer, Department of Clinical Pharmacology, Ninewells Hospital,
Dundee, Scotland

Series Editor:
John L. Reid, MD, FRCP
Regius Professor of Materia Medica, University of Glasgow, Scotland

ISBN-13: 978-3-540-19504-7   e-ISBN-13: 978-1-4471-3145-8
DOI: 10.1007/978-1-4471-3145-8

British Library Cataloguing in Publication Data
Feek, Colin
Endocrine and metabolic disease. – (Treatment in clinical medicine).
1. Endocrine glands – Diseases – Treatment I. Title II. Edwards, Christopher
III. Series 616.4′06   RC649

Library of Congress Cataloging-in-Publication Data
Feek, Colin M. (Colin Michael), 1949 –
Endocrine and metabolic disease. (Treatment in clinical medicine)
Bibliography: p. Includes index.
1. Endocrine glands – Diseases – Treatment. 2. Metabolism – Disorders –
Treatment. I. Edwards, C. R. W. (Christopher Richard Watkin) II. Struthers,
Allan D. III. Title. IV. Series. [DNLM: 1. Endocrine Diseases – therapy. 2.
Endocrine Glands – physiology. 3. Metabolic Diseases – therapy. WK 100 F295e]
RC648.F44   1987   616.4   87–28783

Filmset by Wilmaset, Birkenhead, Merseyside
Printed by Henry Ling, The Dorset Press, Dorchester

2128/3916 543210

For William, Richard and Sam

Series Editor's Foreword

Endocrine and Metabolic Disease is the seventh book in a series of monographs on "Treatment in Clinical Medicine". Each book is complete in its own right and has been prepared by practising physicians with an interest in treatment and management, together with scientists involved in clinical research. The volumes are intended to fill a gap between standard textbooks of medicine and therapeutics and research reviews, symposia and original articles in superspecialist fields. It is the aim of the series to give authoritative up-to-date advice on treatment and management which will be of use to both specialists and non-specialists, and to allow recent advances in pathophysiology and developments in treatment to be viewed in the context of contemporary clinical practice. The approach is intentionally didactic. Each volume has been written by a minimum number of authors to ensure a degree of continuity and uniformity of style. The authors of this volume are Christopher Edwards and Colin Feek. They are widely respected clinical endocrinologists. Christopher Edwards is Professor of Clinical Medicine at the Western General Hospital, University of Edinburgh and Colin Feek, now a specialist physician in endocrinology in Wellington, New Zealand, was formerly a lecturer in Medicine at Edinburgh University. The book is based on their extensive clinical experience and research interests in endocrinology and metabolism.

As with previous volumes in the series, this book is divided into two sections. The first section systematically reviews clinical and therapeutic aspects of endocrine diseases, while the second section considers the clinical pharmacology of drugs used in endocrinology. All the major areas of endocrinology and metabolism are covered. The major fields of thyroid, adrenal and pancreatic disease are covered in depth and there are separate chapters on the ovary and testes, as well as on the pituitary gland and parathyroids. Allan Struthers, Senior Lecturer in Clinical Pharmacology at the University of Dundee, has contributed a chapter on the Clinical Pharmacology of Endocrine Drugs and there is a useful pharmacopoeia of drugs used in endocrinology included at the end of the volume.

This book should be useful to a wide range of doctors, medical students and other health personnel. It does not deal exclusively with rare syndromes but emphasises a practical approach to common clinical problems in endocrinology and metabolism.

Glasgow, November 1987   John L. Reid

Preface

The last decade has seen a major revolution in the development of endocrinology. In particular, the development of radioimmunoassays for hormones in biological fluids has improved our understanding of endocrinology in both health and disease, and their ready availability in the routine market-place of clinical medicine has permitted a greater accuracy of diagnosis. Advances in surgical technique have included the combination of the operating microscope and image intensifier for transsphenoidal surgery in the treatment of pituitary tumours, offering an operation with a high success rate and little morbidity. In the case of prolactin-secreting tumours, however, the advent of dopamine agonist therapy, achieving shrinkage of macroadenomas with restoration of vision where optic pathways have been involved, means that these patients can be treated without the urgent intervention of a skilled neurosurgeon. Computers are increasingly being used in the routine follow-up of common endocrine conditions, such as thyroid disease, allowing effective surveillance of a large reservoir of patients and response to changes in their hormonal status. Recombinant DNA technology has ensured supplies of pure human insulin and human growth hormone.

The object of this book is to present the current treatment of endocrine disease in the light of our latest understanding of endocrine physiology, the natural history of endocrine disorders and the therapeutic options available. We have tried to put the success of these various regimens into some perspective and to indicate those areas of endocrinology where current therapy is either unsatisfactory or without effect. In many of these, such as the disabling and lethal complications of diabetes and osteoporosis, there is obviously a great need for further research.

We are indebted to Allan Struthers for his contribution on the clinical pharmacology of endocrine drugs. We would also like to thank Kevin Miller for producing the illustrations for this book, and Alison Munro for her help in typing and proofreading the manuscript.

July 1987   Colin M. Feek
                        Christopher R. W. Edwards

Contents

SECTION I
Systematic Review of Endocrine Diseases

1 The Thyroid Gland

Thyroid disease is the commonest endocrine disorder. The hormones secreted by the thyroid, thyroxine (T_4) and triiodothyronine (T_3), are regulated by anterior pituitary secretion of thyrotrophin (TSH). TSH stimulates not only function but also growth of the thyroid gland. This is mediated through two different regions of the TSH receptor so that function and growth are usually coupled together. In its turn TSH is regulated by the hypothalamic secretion of thyrotrophin-releasing hormone (TRH).

The synthesis of thyroid hormones is in three steps; active transport of iodide into thyroid cells, intracellular oxidation of iodide to iodine and iodination of tyrosyl residues within thyroglobulin (Fig. 1.1). There are approximately 120 tyrosyl residues in the thyroglobulin molecule and the proportion of monoiodotyrosines to diiodotyrosines determines the relative quantity of T_4 to T_3 synthesised. This is approximately 10:1, but changes in iodine deficiency, with greater production of T_3. Thyroglobulin is synthesised in the thyroid cell and after undergoing iodination it is stored in the follicular fluid by a process of exocytosis. Thyroid hormones are released from intrafollicular thyroglobulin by endocytosis and subsequent proteolysis in the thyroid cell to yield thyroglobulin, T_4 and T_3. Thyroglobulin reaches the general circulation from the thyroid lymphatics, and serum concentrations of thyroglobulin are controlled by TSH. The thyroid secretes approximately 70–90 µg of T_4 and 15–30 µg of T_3 per day, but only 20% of plasma T_3 is derived from direct thyroidal secretion. Eighty per cent of plasma T_3 is derived by conversion from T_4.

T_4 is a prohormone that is converted in peripheral tissues (liver, kidney and brain) either to the active hormone T_3 or to biologically inactive reverse T_3 (rT_3). This is achieved by the enzyme monodeiodinase which exists in two forms. Type I is localised to liver and kidney; its activity is decreased by hypothyroidism, increased by hyperthyroidism and inhibited by propyl-thiouracil. The enzyme is responsible for the majority of circulating T_3. In

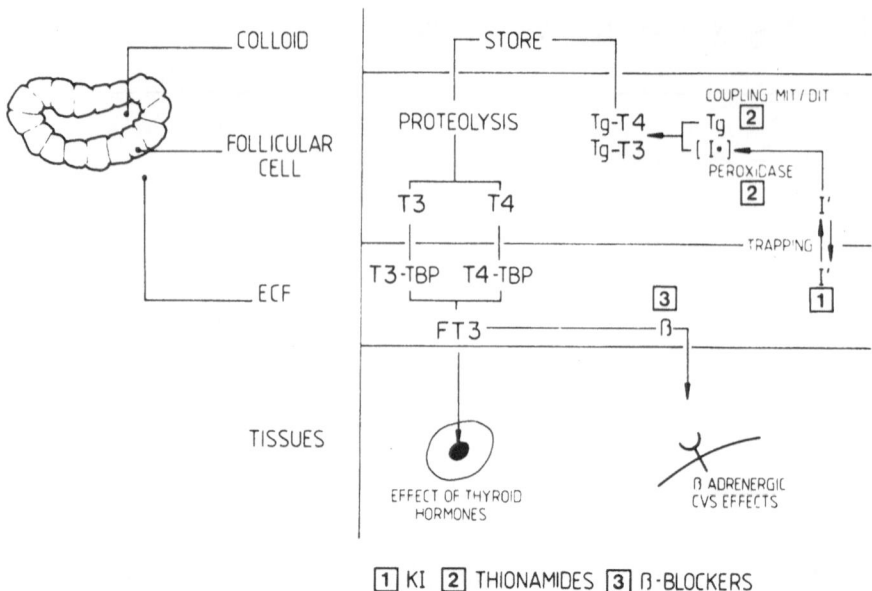

Fig. 1.1. The major steps of and sites of action of potassium iodide (KI), thionamides and β-adrenoceptor blocking drugs upon the biosynthesis of thyroid hormones. (CVS, cardiovascular system; FT_3, free T_3; I, iodine; MIT/DIT, mono- and diiodotyrosines; Tg, thyroglobulin; TBP, thyroid-binding proteins.)

contrast, type II is localised to the brain; its activity is increased by hypothyroidism and decreased by hyperthyroidism and it provides T_3 direct to cells. Liver and kidney derive approximately 80% of T_3 from the blood and 20% from local production whereas the converse is true for the brain. The physiological consequence of this is to protect the brain against hypothyroidism by decreasing the amount of T_4 converted by liver and kidney to T_3 to supply the blood, reserving T_4 for local conversion to T_3 by the brain. Peripheral conversion of T_4 to active T_3 is inhibited by non-thyroidal illness, glucocorticoids, β-adrenoceptor blocking drugs, amiodarone, sodium ipodate (a radiological contrast agent) and propylthiouracil, with increased formation of biologically inactive rT_3. In the circulation T_4 is bound to a specific protein, thyroxine-binding globulin (TBG), and to a lesser extent thyroxine-binding pre-albumin. These transport proteins are synthesised by the liver.

Thyroid hormones exert effects on a great multiplicity of metabolic processes. They stimulate calorigenesis with an associated increase in oxygen consumption possibly as a result of the energy released from stimulation of the Na-K–ATPase enzyme.

These hormones also stimulate protein synthesis and are required in adequate amounts for the synthesis and secretion of growth hormone. However, thyroid hormones in excess may inhibit protein synthesis and increase the concentration of free amino acids in plasma, liver and muscle. They act on carbohydrate metabolism by potentiating the effects of insulin on glycogen synthesis and glucose utilisation. However, thyroid hormones also increase the degradation of insulin so that diminished sensitivity to administered insulin may occur in hyperthyroidism with the converse in hypothyroidism. They also appear to regulate the glycogenolytic and hyperglycaemic actions of catecholamines. The action of thyroid hormones on the sympatho-adrenal system is to increase the sensitivity of tissues to catecholamines by "up-regulation" of β-adrenoceptors involving increased number, increased coupling of the receptor and increased adenylate cyclase activity. As regards lipid metabolism thyroid hormones appear to stimulate synthesis, mobilisation and degradation, but as degradation is stimulated more than synthesis the net result is to decrease the stores and plasma levels of most lipids including triglycerides, phospholipids and cholesterol.

Lastly, thyroid hormones increase the demand for coenzymes and the vitamins from which they are derived. In hyperthyroidism, the requirements for water-soluble vitamins such as thiamine, riboflavin, B_{12} and vitamin C are increased with resulting reductions in tissue concentrations. The same is true for the fat-soluble vitamins A, D and E. The action of thyroid hormones at the cellular level is to enhance substrate availability at the plasma membrane, to provide metabolic energy for the mitochondria and to direct synthesis of specific structural and functional components of the cell at the transcriptional and post-transcriptional level.

Thyroid hormones are routinely measured by radioimmunoassay and the results reflect the plasma total thyroid hormone levels (bound as well as free), not the biologically active free fraction. The free thyroxine index (FT_4I) is still calculated by many laboratories as an indirect estimate of free thyroxine but is gradually being superseded by methods that estimate free hormones directly. Non-thyroidal illness such as pneumonia, myocardial infarction and diabetic ketoacidosis is being increasingly recognised as causing a variety of abnormalities of thyroid function. Three basic patterns of change in plasma thyroid hormone concentrations occur. Common to all three is a decrease in plasma total T_3 with a concomitant rise in plasma rT_3 concentrations due to impaired peripheral conversion of T_4 to T_3.

1. In the first category, impaired peripheral conversion results in an increase in both plasma free and total T_4 and a normal or slightly raised plasma TSH. (Regulation of TSH secretion by the thyrotrophs is mediated by the intrapituitary conversion of T_4 to T_3.) The implication of this finding in non-thyroidal illness is that a raised plasma free T_4 does not therefore necessarily mean that the patient is hyperthyroid. However, a low plasma free T_4 usually equates with hypothyroidism.

2. In the second category, plasma free T_4 is increased as before but plasma total T_4 is decreased as a result of impaired synthesis of thyroxine-binding pre-albumin.

3. In the third category, plasma free T_4 levels are elevated but plasma total T_4 falls to an undetectable level. This usually occurs in severe illness. The fall

		1° ATROPHIC HYPOTHYROIDISM	HASHIMOTO'S THYROIDITIS	GRAVES' DISEASE	SIMPLE/MULTI NODULAR GOITRE
GOITRE		−	+++	− to +++	+++
STATUS		HYPOTHYROID	HYPO TO HYPERTHYROID	HYPERTHYROID	EU – HYPERTHYROID
ANTIBODIES					
CYTOPLASM/COLLOID		++	+++	+	±
TSH R Ab	BLOCK	+	+	−	−
	STIMULATE	−	+	+++	±
Growth Ab	BLOCK	+++	−	−	−
	STIMULATE	−	−	− to +++	+++
EXOPHTHALMOS		+	+	+++	−

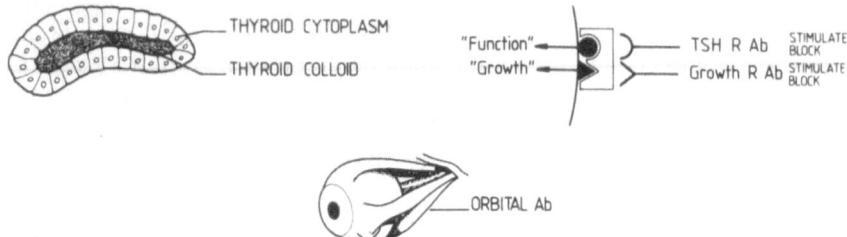

Fig. 1.2. The autoimmune spectrum of thyroid disease in relation to different thyroid autoantibodies. (TSH R Ab, TSH-receptor antibody; Growth R Ab, growth-receptor antibody.)

in plasma total T_4 levels has prognostic implications in relation to subsequent mortality.

It is now clear that the majority of thyroid conditions are the result of autoimmunity. A wide spectrum of autoantibodies (Fig. 1.2) has been described to account for the varied clinical presentation of thyroid disease. Antibodies against thyroid cytoplasm (microsomal antibodies) and thyroid colloid (thyroglobulin antibodies) result in progressive destruction of the gland, which in turn results in hypothyroidism. Antibodies may occupy the portion of the TSH receptor coupled to adenyl cyclase, either blocking or stimulating the secretion of thyroid hormones (TSH-receptor antibodies). Similarly antibodies may occupy the portion of the TSH receptor coupled to growth, either blocking or stimulating goitre formation (growth-receptor antibodies). Thus, in disease, function of the thyroid and growth may be dissociated. Antibodies against a specific orbital antigen (orbital immunoglobulins) are responsible for endocrine exophthalmos. So far, none of these antibodies have been implicated in tumours of the thyroid.

Figure 1.3 outlines a scheme for differentiating the various thyroid conditions and is divided into two steps:

1. What is the patient's thyroid function?

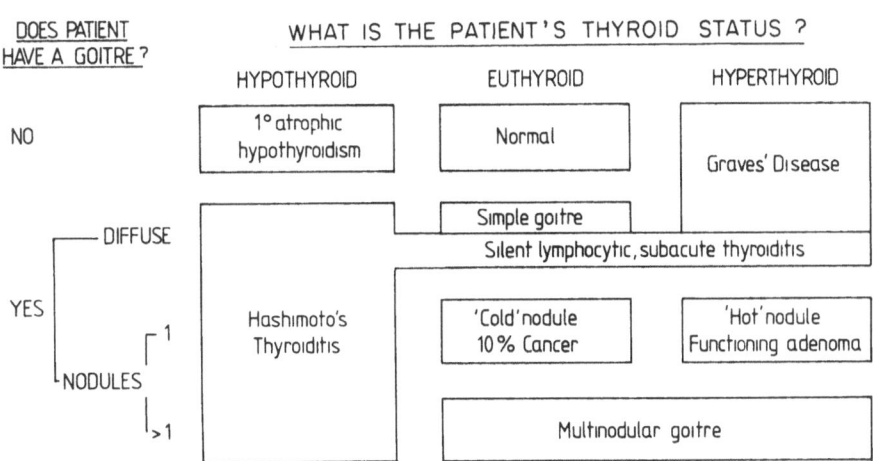

Fig. 1.3. A scheme for differentiating the various disorders of the thyroid gland (see text for details).

2. Is a goitre present? If a goitre is present, palpation and thyroid scintigraphy will determine whether the gland is diffusely enlarged or nodular and the extent of nodularity. ^{99m}Tc-pertechnetate is usually used for scintigraphy (Fig. 1.4). This is trapped by the thyroid in a similar manner to iodine. In addition, lateral and posterior–anterior radiography of the thoracic inlet should be performed to assess any tracheal deviation or compression.

Hypothyroidism

Hypothyroidism is common in the United Kingdom, with a prevalence of overt hypothyroidism of 14 cases per 1000 females and 1 per 1000 males.

Diagnosis

Hypothyroidism with Raised Plasma TSH Levels

Estimation of plasma total T_4 levels alone is insufficient to make a diagnosis of primary hypothyroidism—estimation of plasma TSH is also required. There are two major spontaneous causes:

1. *Hashimoto's thyroiditis* is characterised by the presence of a goitre and a high titre of autoantibodies in the blood against thyroid cytoplasm (micro-

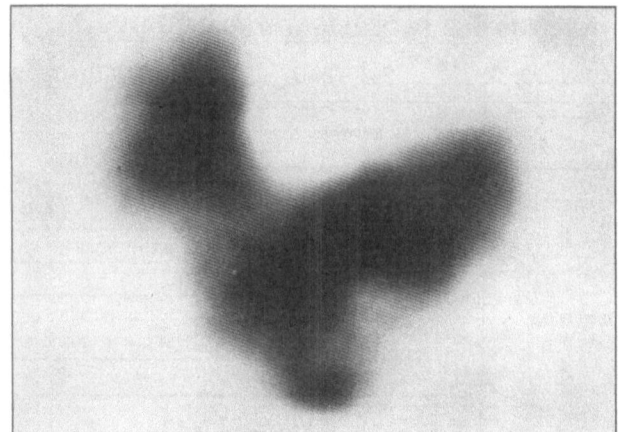

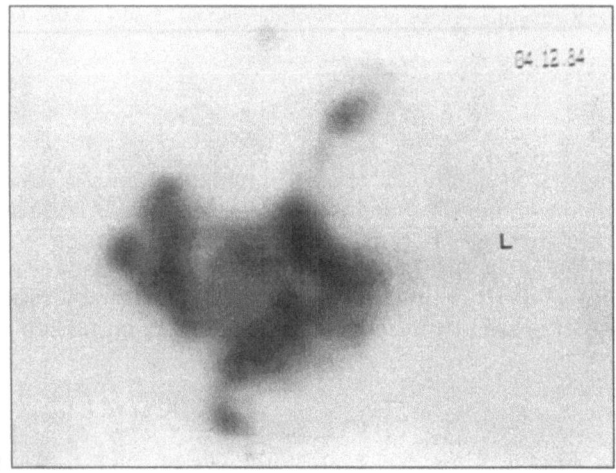

Fig. 1.4. Thyroid scintigraphy using ⁹⁹ᵐTc-pertechnetate to demonstrate a diffuse goitre (**a**), a multinodular goitre (**b**), a "hot" nodule of the isthmus (**c**) and a cold nodule of the *right* lobe (**d**).

somes) and colloid (thyroglobulin). Goitre formation results from compensatory TSH stimulation, lymphocytic infiltration and fibrosis.

2. *Primary atrophic hypothyroidism* differs from Hashimoto's thyroiditis in the absence of a goitre and in less elevated titres of thyroid autoantibodies. Goitre formation resulting from compensatory TSH stimulation is inhibited by an antibody (growth-receptor-blocking antibody).

These two conditions account for the majority of cases. Other causes include radioiodine and drug or surgical treatment for hyperthyroidism, iodide deficiency, dyshormonogenesis and thyroid agenesis. Routine screen-

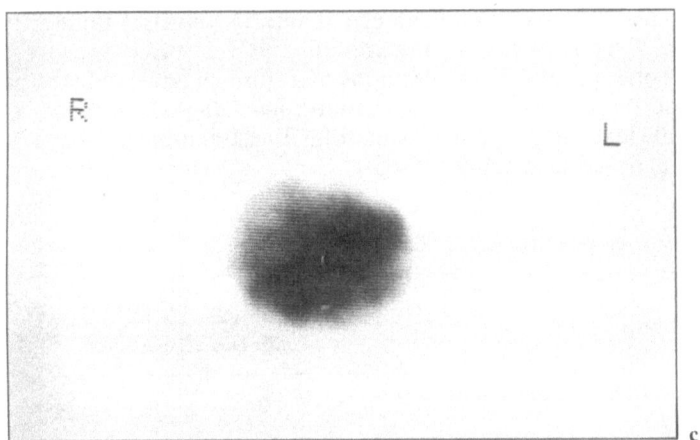

c

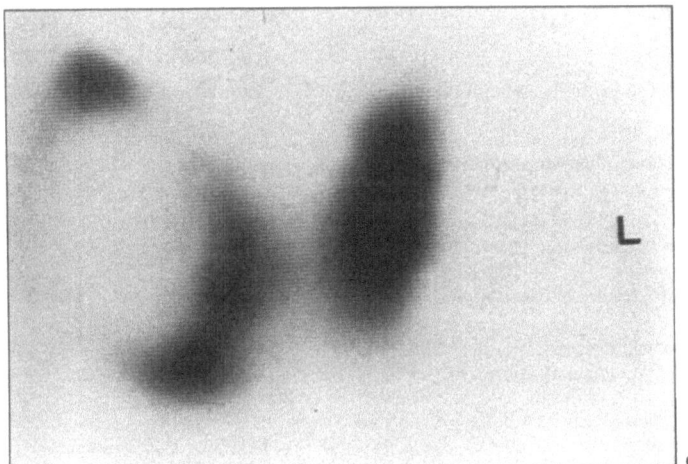

d

ing of capillary blood spots for TSH estimation, 5–7 days after birth, has demonstrated an incidence of congenital hypothyroidism of 1 in 4000 births, making it possible to carry out early treatment and thus prevent irreversible brain damage.

Hypothyroidism with Normal or Low Plasma TSH Levels

A diagnosis of secondary (pituitary or hypothalamic) hypothyroidism is suspected on the basis of low plasma total T_4 and low TSH levels. Patients with this condition usually have other evidence of anterior pituitary failure. In these patients the TSH response to intravenous TRH is often preserved despite subnormal plasma total T_4 levels and is therefore an unreliable test in this condition. Non-thyroidal illness, renal failure, liver disease, a variety of drugs and TBG deficiency may lower plasma total T_4 estimations (Table 1.1) and may be misdiagnosed as pituitary disease.

Table 1.1. Factors interfering with thyroid function and in vitro thyroid function tests

	T_4		T_3		TSH
	Total	Free	Total	Free	
Factors causing low total serum T_4 concentrations					
Illness					
1. Non-thyroidal illness: myocardial infarct, pneumonia	↓	N	↓	↓	N
2. Chronic renal failure	↓	N	↓	↓	Nᵃ
3. Chronic liver disease	↓	N	↓	↓ N	N ↑
Drugs					
1. Inhibitors of thyroid hormone synthesis: lithium, sulphonamides, sulphonylureas, p-aminosalicylic acid, phenylbutazone	↓	↓	↓	↓	↑
2. Altered binding to TBG: phenytoin, salicylates, feclofenac, phenylbutazone	↓	N	↓	↓	N
3. Acceleration of T_4 metabolism: phenytoin, glucocorticoidsᵇ	↓	↓	N	N	N
Factors causing elevated total serum T_4 and T_3 concentrations					
Thyroxine and triiodothyronine autoantibodies	↑	Nᶜ	↑	Nᶜ	N
Drugs					
1. Stimulation of thyroid hormone synthesis: iodide	↑	↑	↑	↑	↓
2. Increased serum TBG concentrations: oestrogen, pregnancy, clofibrate	↑	N	↑	N	N
3. Interference with peripheral metabolism of thyroid hormones: amiodarone, iopanoic acid	↑	↑	↓	↓	↑

ᵃBlunted response to TRH.
ᵇSuppressed pituitary secretion of TSH to TRH.
ᶜAfter appropriate separation from serum.

Treatment

Primary hypothyroidism is treated by the oral administration of L-thyroxine. It is given once a day and has a half-life of 6.7 days. In chronic hypothyroidism, developing in patients without any evidence of ischaemic heart disease, it is usual to start by giving 50 µg daily, increasing the dose by 50 µg at 2- weekly intervals until full replacement is achieved. This is usually 100–200 µg daily. Full replacement is assessed by biochemical results after 3 months of treatment. Plasma TSH estimations before this period are not a true reflection of TSH status because of pituitary thyrotroph hyperplasia following a sustained period of hypothyroidism. L-Thyroxine can be prescribed in different strengths: 25, 50 or 100 μg. Unfortunately they are not colour-coded and errors result from incorrect identification of tablet strengths. It is wise to ask the patient to bring the bottle of thyroid pills with them so that the dose of thyroxine can be checked.

The plasma total T_4 levels achieved by L-thyroxine administration sufficient to suppress plasma TSH levels to within the normal range is higher than the upper limit of the normal reference range. Many laboratories quote a different reference range for patients receiving thyroxine. In addition the ratio of T_4 to T_3 differs from normal, being increased as a result of loss of thyroidal secretion of T_3, first pass metabolism through the liver and autoregulation of conversion of T_4 to T_3 (the efficiency of monodeiodination decreases as plasma total T_4 rises). Drugs such as cholestyramine may interfere with the absorption of L-thyroxine.

Care must be taken in instituting replacement in those patients with ischaemic heart disease. Angina or sudden death may be precipitated. In such patients replacement with triiodothyronine may be useful as the drug has a shorter half-life than thyroxine and can be easily discontinued if angina is precipitated. It is usual to start with low doses (2.5–5 μg 8-hourly), increased gradually to 10 μg 8-hourly over a period of a week. If the patient is stable on this dose, treatment with L-thyroxine can be started at a dose of 100 μg daily and the oral triiodothyronine withdrawn after a 3-day overlap. Treatment must be supervised in hospital with regular electrocardiographic monitoring. If angina is severe enough to prevent the institution of full replacement therapy despite the administration of β-adrenoceptor blocking drugs, coronary angiography should be considered prior to coronary artery by-pass surgery in suitable patients. Following this procedure the thyroxine dose can usually be increased to optimal replacement. In patients who have been rendered acutely hypothyroid as a result of recent radioiodine treatment or surgery, it is not necessary to introduce replacement therapy gradually: full replacement therapy (150–200 μg daily) should be initiated as soon as possible.

L-Thyroxine is used to treat Hashimoto's thyroiditis if the patient is hypothyroid but it can also be considered if the patient is euthyroid in an attempt to shrink the goitre. This can be achieved if there is little fibrosis and lymphocyte infiltrate.

Hyperthyroidism

Hyperthyroidism is common in the United Kingdom, with a prevalence of overt hyperthyroidism in 20 per 1000 females and 2 per 1000 males.

Diagnosis

Hyperthyroidism with Suppressed Plasma TSH Levels

Plasma total T_4 is clearly elevated in more than 90% of patients with primary hyperthyroidism. It may be normal, however, in some patients who have T_3 thyrotoxicosis. Plasma total T_3 levels may be normal or low in patients with hyperthyroidism and coexisting non-thyroidal illness such as heart failure. When a diagnosis of hyperthyroidism is in doubt it is usual to assess the plasma TSH response to the intravenous administration of TRH 200 μg. However this is now being superseded by the introduction of immuno-radiometric assays (IRMA) for TSH with low levels of detection that can differentiate normal from suppressed plasma TSH concentrations.

Once the diagnosis of hyperthyroidism is established, the thyroidal radioiodine uptake is determined over a specified period either after the oral administration of ^{131}I (4 hours) or more conveniently after the intravenous administration of ^{99m}Tc-pertechnetate (20 minutes). The uptake is high in the three main causes of hyperthyroidism:

1. *Graves' disease* is caused by TSH-receptor antibody which stimulates thyroid hormone secretion by stimulating the portion of the TSH receptor that is coupled to adenyl cyclase in a similar manner to TSH. Patients may develop a diffuse goitre if growth-receptor antibodies are present, exophthalmos if orbital-stimulating immunoglobulins are present and pretibial myx-oedema.

2. *Multinodular goitre* is an ill-understood disorder but thyroid growth is probably stimulated by a growth-receptor-stimulating antibody. Growth of new follicles outstrips local blood supply resulting in necrosis in the centre of growth, followed by repair and fibrosis with the formation of multiple nodules. The intensity of the stimulus to growth is relatively weak in multinodular goitre when compared with TSH and its receptor antibody.

It appears that the basic event in thyroid growth is multiplication of epithelial cells within the follicular wall (Fig. 1.5). This process eventually leads to either enlargement of the follicle or the generation of new follicles by the development of daughter follicle buds. Epithelial cells of a mother follicle are heterogeneous for characteristics of growth and function, whereas epithelial cells of daughter follicles are monoclonal, generated from a single cell of the mother follicle. Thus a mother follicle has the potential of generating new follicles of differing levels of growth and function. Moreover the potential for growth is not necessarily related to function so that follicles created from a mother follicle may vary in their capacity to iodinate thyroglobulin—one may be "**hot**" whilst the other is "**cold**".

In the presence of a weak growth stimulator alone, only those scattered cells in maternal follicles with high growth potential are selected to form new daughter follicles that vary in their shape, size and function. Over the years there is a relentless formation of new follicles with widely varying metabolic activity. In contrast, in the presence of a strong combined stimulator of

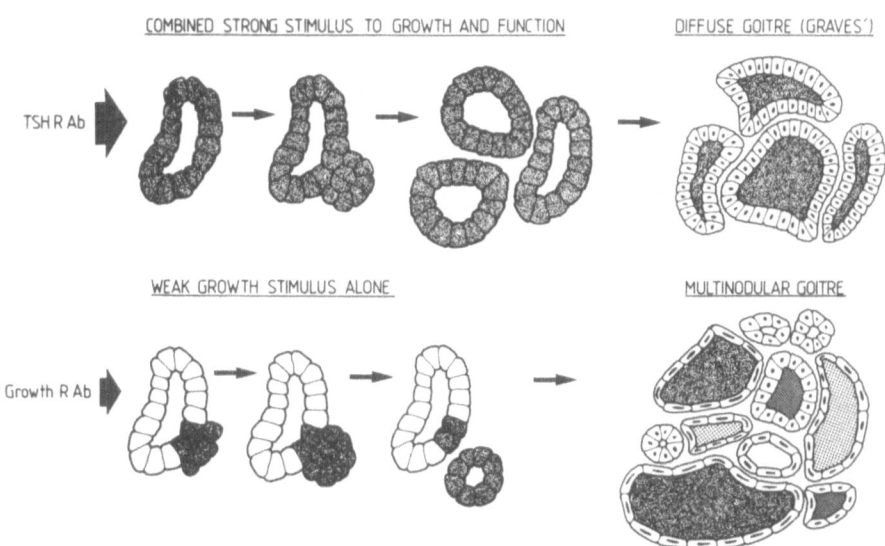

COMBINED STRONG STIMULUS TO GROWTH AND FUNCTION   DIFFUSE GOITRE (GRAVES')

TSH R Ab

WEAK GROWTH STIMULUS ALONE   MULTINODULAR GOITRE

Growth R Ab

Fig. 1.5. In the presence of a combined stimulus to growth and function, such as TSH or its receptor antibody (TSH R Ab), all cells within the thyroid follicle are stimulated to produce daughter follicles and a goitre characterised by follicles of the same size and the same type of high columnar epithelium, and all cells have the same iodine turnover (Graves' disease). In the presence of a weak growth stimulus alone, such as growth-receptor-stimulating antibody (Growth R Ab), only a few sensitive cells within the follicle are stimulated to produce daughter follicles and a goitre characterised by follicles of various sizes, epithelial height and iodine turnover (multinodular goitre).

growth and function, TSH or its receptor antibody, follicles are formed which are alike and display intense metabolic activity (Fig. 1.5).

3. *Autonomous thyroid adenomas* are benign well-differentiated tumours that secrete excessive amounts of thyroid hormones. On thyroid scintigraphy the palpable nodule is "hot" with suppression of the surrounding normal gland.

Radioiodine uptake is subnormal in some uncommon causes of hyperthyroidism which are thus not candidates for destructive therapy.

1. *Silent lymphocytic thyroiditis* is a condition which is being diagnosed with increasing frequency, accounting for up to 20% of cases of hyperthyroidism in North America. It is characterised by a diffuse painless goitre and the lack of other stigmata seen in patients with Graves' disease. Serum thyroid autoantibodies are positive during the active phase and thyroid aspiration yields many lymphocytes. The course proceeds spontaneously from hyper- to hypothyroidism with full recovery in 3 or 6 months. The hyperthyroid phase is a direct result of the release of thyroid hormones and thyroglobulin into the blood by the intense thyroiditis. The hypothyroid phase results from

depletion of intrathyroidal thyroid hormone stores; euthyroidism follows as thyroid hormone synthesis is restored.

2. *Subacute (DeQuervain's) thyroiditis* is a self-limiting form of hyperthyroidism similar to silent lymphocytic thyroiditis but is established as a distinct entity by the finding of a painful goitre with infiltration by neutrophils and macrophages, microabscess formation, necrosis and multinucleated giant cells. The disorder is probably viral in aetiology with a clinical course similar to silent lymphocytic thyroiditis.

Other causes of hyperthyroidism with a suppressed uptake are thyrotoxicosis factitia, Jod Basedow and struma ovarii.

Hyperthyroidism with Normal or Raised Plasma TSH Levels

This occurs extremely rarely in two situations:

1. *TSH-secreting pituitary tumours* in which plasma TSH levels fail to respond to the intravenous administration of TRH, fail to suppress in response to the administration of L-thyroxine and in which the inappropriate secretion of TSH is associated with increased secretion of α-subunit (the glycopeptides TSH, FSH and LH share a common α-subunit with a different β-subunit conferring biological and immunological specificity). In approximately two-thirds of cases isolated TSH hypersecretion is found, but in one-third TSH secretion is associated with excess secretion of GH and/or prolactin. Patients have classical features of hyperthyroidism, goitre but no evidence of exophthalmos. A pituitary microadenoma is usually demonstrated by computerised tomography.

2. *Pituitary resistance to the action of thyroid hormones* is another cause of inappropriate TSH secretion, resulting in elevation of plasma thyroid hormone levels, goitre and hyperthyroidism. These patients differ from those with a TSH-secreting pituitary tumour in responsiveness of plasma TSH levels to the administration of TRH and suppression following the administration of L-thyroxine. Where resistance to thyroid hormones exists not only in the anterior pituitary but also in peripheral tissues, the patient will develop elevated plasma thyroid hormone levels, goitre and either compensated euthyroidism or hypothyroidism.

Other factors causing elevation of plasma total thyroid hormone levels are shown in Table 1.1.

Treatment

Whatever the underlying condition there are certain general measures that should be employed. The majority of patients can be treated as outpatients. Associated cardiac failure should be treated with an appropriate diuretic, and atrial fibrillation with digoxin. Anticoagulation therapy should be considered if atrial fibrillation is present because of the risk, albeit small, of cerebral embolism. Elective cardioversion should be postponed until the patient is euthyroid.

Hyperthyroidism may be effectively treated by one method or a combination of three methods:

1. *Antithyroid drugs* in common use are the thionamides—carbimazole and propylthiouracil. These drugs act by inhibiting the incorporation of iodide into the tyrosine residues of thyroglobulin and subsequent coupling of mono- and diiodotyrosines which normally leads to thyroid hormone synthesis (Fig. 1.1). In addition, propylthiouracil interferes with the peripheral conversion of T_4 to T_3. Treatment with antithyroid drugs is an easy and effective method of controlling hyperthyroidism but relapse will occur on drug withdrawal if the underlying stimulus to hyperthyroidism is still present.

Carbimazole is metabolised to methimazole before it is biologically active and is conventionally prescribed in doses of 45–60 mg per day initially, reducing to a maintenance dose of 10 mg per day when the patient has been rendered euthyroid. However, carbimazole has been shown to be equally effective when given in a lower initial dose of 20 mg per day, irrespective of the severity of hyperthyroidism; the dose is reduced once the patient is euthyroid (after approximately 6 weeks). Despite the fact that plasma half-life of carbimazole is short (4–6 hours) the biological effect lasts longer (up to 40 hours) so that patients may be treated with once-daily doses.

The dose of the drug should be titrated by its clinical effect coupled with serial estimation of plasma total T_4 and T_3. Once control is achieved the patient should receive the lowest dose of drug to maintain euthyroidism. Patients treated with carbimazole should be warned that 5% may develop a skin rash and 0.05%–0.3% agranulocytosis. This may be heralded by a sore throat. Monitoring neutrophil counts routinely is no help but should be performed immediately if agranulocytosis is suspected. The cause of agranulocytosis is unknown but the association with anti-neutrophil antibodies suggests an autoimmune phenomenon rather than bone marrow toxicity. The risk of agranulocytosis with carbimazole is dose-related. Methimazole is not significantly bound by plasma proteins, unlike propylthiouracil which is extensively bound to plasma albumin.

Propylthiouracil is therefore prescribed in larger doses than carbimazole, initially 450–600 mg, reducing to 100 mg per day. The plasma half-life (1.5 hours) and biological half-life (considerably less than 40 hours) of propylthiouracil are shorter than those of methimazole, making once-daily doses less effective. Therefore, all things being equal, carbimazole 20 mg once daily is the preferred drug of choice unless the patient is allergic to carbimazole or is breast-feeding.

The administration of a β-adrenoceptor blocking drug such as propranolol is useful to block the sympathomimetic action of thyroid hormones (Fig. 1.1) and, when given acutely impairs the peripheral conversion of T_4 to T_3. It is important to remember that the other metabolic consequences of thyroid hormone excess continue unaffected and this may prevent the successful use of propranolol in some patients. Propranolol-LA is given in a dose of 160 mg once daily by mouth, providing there is no contraindication.

Potassium iodide is an antithyroid drug acting by inhibition of the synthesis and release of thyroid hormones (Fig. 1.1). It has long been recognised that not all patients with hyperthyroidism respond satisfactorily, and that in some the use of iodide may exacerbate thyrotoxicosis. Furthermore the effect of iodide is transient and a secondary rise in plasma thyroid hormone levels may occur after 10 days of treatment. The use of iodide is therefore restricted to the preparation of patients for thyroid surgery where it may be used in combination with a β-adrenoceptor blocking drug (Fig. 1.6). The addition of potassium iodide (60 mg 8-hourly) to propranolol unfortunately eliminates the flexibility of the timing of the operation.

2. The aim of *surgery* is to remove the bulk of the thyroid gland (subtotal thyroidectomy) leaving a remnant to maintain normal thyroid hormone secretion. There is some evidence to suggest that thyroid autoantibodies are synthesised from intrathyroidal lymphocytes and surgery may therefore

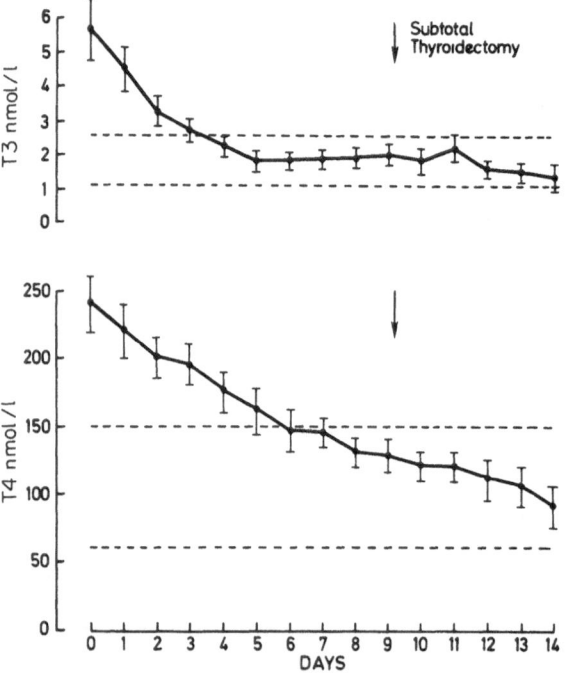

Fig. 1.6. The effect of taking potassium iodide (180 mg/day plus propranolol 160 mg/day) for 10 days before subtotal thyroidectomy on plasma T_4 and T_3 levels in 10 patients with Graves' disease who were already taking propranolol.

remove the stimulus to hyperthyroidism. This form of treatment requires a surgeon who regularly practises neck surgery otherwise morbidity of the operation will be high. Patients are rendered euthyroid prior to surgery by the administration of carbimazole. This can increase plasma TSH levels and the vascularity of the gland. Some centres overcome this problem by combining thionamide therapy with the administration of L-thyroxine to suppress TSH secretion.

Other centres have adopted propranolol as the sole drug in the preparation of patients for thyroid surgery. It has the advantages of shorter preparation time, flexible timing of operation and reduction in operative blood loss. However, the successful use of propranolol requires a high standard of supervision ensuring that no patient is operated upon until the resting pulse rate is less than 90 per minute and that in no case is the important preoperative dose of propranolol omitted on the day of operation. Following surgery, plasma total T_3 levels fall to within the normal range at 1 day and plasma total T_4 levels at 4 days. Propranolol needs to be continued to cover this period. Postoperative hypocalcaemia is common (17%) in propranolol-prepared patients. It occurs particularly in those with an elevated bone plasma alkaline phosphatase and is caused by calcium entry into bones as plasma thyroid hormone levels are restored to normal. Hypocalcaemia may also result from temporary parathyroid damage but permanent hypoparathyroidism occurs in less than 1%. Vocal cord palsy is a complication in 2% and cord movement should be assessed before and after operation. Death unfortunately can occur even in the most experienced hands (less than 1 in 1000 operations).

3. *Radioiodine* is easy to administer but hypothyroidism is a major complication. There has been great concern that the radiation dose to the gonad following the administration of radioiodine to fertile patients may cause genetic damage as well as increase the risk of developing leukaemia or thyroid cancer. The risk of genetic damage assuming a dose of 370 MBq ^{131}I has been estimated to be in the order of 5 per 100 000 live births based on a calculated gonadal dose of 32 mSv. The spontaneous rate is 800 per 100 000. An accumulation of experience in the use of radioiodine in over 1 million patients in North America has failed to demonstrate a discernible genetic risk in the first generation of offspring born to radioiodine-treated patients. There also appears to be no risk of thyroid malignancy or leukaemia.

Selection of appropriate treatment depends on the underlying disorder.

1. *Graves' disease.* Carbimazole is a weak immunosuppressant but does not seem significantly to alter the natural history of the disorder. Approximately 30% of patients presenting with Graves' disease for the first time will enter remission spontaneously within 6–12 months but 70% will run a relapsing–remitting course for the foreseeable future. It is appropriate to treat the first group with thionamides and to submit the second group to destructive treatment. This policy requires some method of prediction. It was hoped that this could be achieved using a combination of HLA typing and estimation of

TSH-receptor antibody in the blood, but encouraging preliminary results have not been substantiated. Antithyroid drugs should be given to children, pregnant women and young adults, reserving destructive therapy for adults over the age of 25 years and those patients who relapse after a course of antithyroid medication. A course of treatment should be limited to 6–12 months as there is little evidence that more prolonged administration is of additional benefit.

Surgery in skilled hands offers an 80% chance of cure, with 6% recurrent hyperthyroidism and 14% hypothyroidism.

Radioiodine therapy is now becoming the treatment of choice where destruction of the thyroid is being contemplated. Over 95% of patients will respond to treatment with this form of therapy. Initially, 370 MBq ^{131}I is given by mouth and the dose is doubled if the patient's symptoms have not been controlled within 6 months. In the 1st year 40%–90% become hypothyroid with a subsequent failure rate of 2.8% per annum (Fig. 1.7). A policy is currently evolving of deliberately rendering patients hypothyroid and subsequently instituting replacement therapy with L-thyroxine. Such a scheme requires lifelong monitoring of patients to ensure compliance with replacement therapy. This can be achieved by regional computerisation, with less than 6% of patients lost to follow-up after 10 years. Over 10% of patients will need adjustments in their replacement therapy during this period.

Some special measures apply to hyperthyroidism arising in pregnancy. Approximately 1 in 1000 pregnancies is complicated by hyperthyroidism.

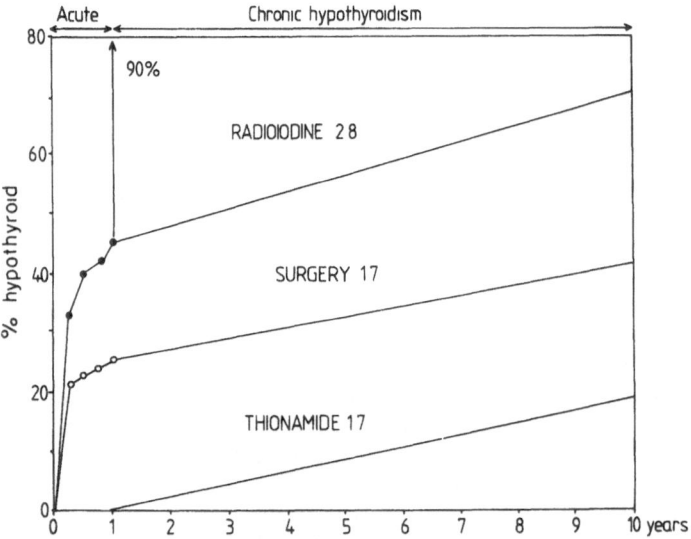

Fig. 1.7. The cumulative incidence (% per year) of hypothyroidism in patients with Graves' disease treated either by antithyroid drugs, surgery or radioiodine.

Antithyroid drugs are the treatment of choice although surgery may be indicated for pregnant women in whom a large goitre may be causing local pressure symptoms or in those who require high doses of carbimazole to render them euthyroid. Carbimazole crosses the placenta and the lowest dose must be employed to maintain maternal euthyroidism if fetal hypothyroidism is to be avoided. Intrauterine hypothyroidism can lead to fetal brain damage. Unlike carbimazole, maternal thyroid hormones do not cross the placenta and there is no place for giving a combination of antithyroid drugs and L-thyroxine. It is essential to titrate the dose of carbimazole to maintain normal maternal plasma thyroid hormone levels. In normal pregnancy there is a marked increase in plasma TBG levels, elevating plasma total T_4 and T_3 estimations. Pregnant patients are best monitored biochemically by the estimation of plasma total T_4, T_3, free thyroid hormones and plasma TSH levels. Radioiodine is obviously contraindicated in pregnancy as is the administration of any other isotope or unnecessary drug. Estimation of maternal serum TSH-receptor antibody towards the end of pregnancy and fetal cardiotocography may predict the risk or detect the development of fetal hyperthyroidism which can be treated by administration of a β-adrenoceptor blocking drug either to the mother or to the newborn infant until maternal TSH-receptor antibody is cleared from the fetal circulation following delivery.

It is important to remember that fetal hyperthyroidism can also develop as a result of raised maternal TSH-receptor antibodies in mothers with Graves' disease who have been rendered euthyroid by previous destructive therapy. This situation can be treated by a combination of thyroxine and carbimazole.

Neonatal hypothyroidism is a theoretical risk to breastfed infants of mothers receiving antithyroid medication. However, propylthiouracil being protein-bound is only secreted in small amounts in breast milk and is preferable to carbimazole.

Endocrine exophthalmos occurs most commonly in association with Graves' disease but may also be associated with primary atrophic hypothyroidism, Hashimoto's thyroiditis, and may be seen in patients without obvious thyroid disease. In the latter group plasma thyroid hormones are in the normal reference range but approximately one-third of patients will have an attenuated TSH response to TRH, one-third an exaggerated response and one-third a normal response. The female to male ratio in endocrine exophthalmos is 2:1 compared with 6:1 in Graves' disease alone.

An antibody directed against an orbital antigen causes swelling of the extraocular eye muscles increasing their volume up to 10 times. The average orbital volume is approximately 26 ml and 1 mm proptosis will result from an increase of 0.7 ml. Thus considerable exophthalmos of some 6 mm will be caused by a bulk increase of only 4 ml. The bulk of the muscles is increased by a lymphocytic infiltrate, fat and deposition of mucopolysaccharides which aggravate the problem by a marked propensity to bind water. Increased muscle volume displaces the globe anteriorly (proptosis) and swelling at the orbital cone may compress the optic nerve causing papilloedema and blindness. Inflammation and fibrosis in the muscles causes shortening and

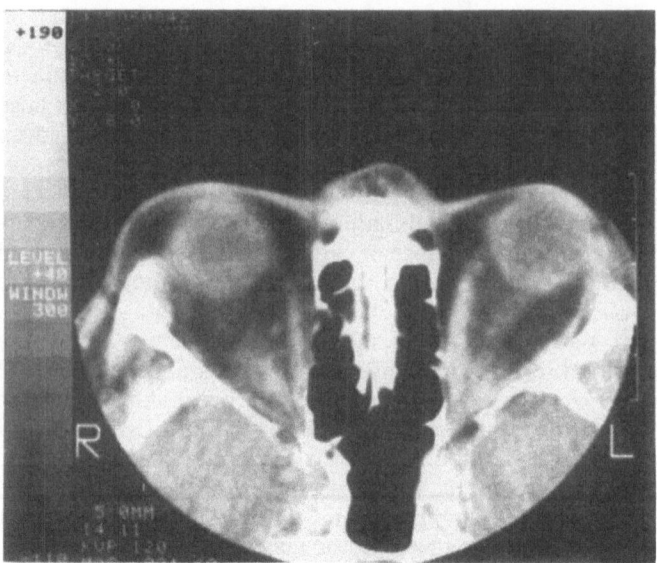

Fig. 1.8. Computerised axial tomography of the orbits of a patient with endocrine exophthalmos. (Courtesy Dr R Sellar, Department of Neuroradiology, Western General Hospital, Edinburgh.)

diplopia. Clinical evaluation, exophthalmometry and computerised axial tomography (Fig. 1.8) are best used to monitor the patient.

Most patients require no treatment. Patients may be divided into two groups—those with mild non-progressive ophthalmopathy and those with severe progressive ophthalmopathy.

In mild ophthalmopathy little or no treatment may be required but "grittiness" may be treated with methylcellulose eye drops (it is important to exclude any corneal abrasions first). Recurrent episodes of corneal damage are an indication for tarsorrhaphy.

Fortunately, severe eye involvement occurs in less than 2% of patients with Graves' disease. Progressive ophthalmopathy producing severe complications from proptosis, diplopia or visual failure should be treated with high-dose corticosteroid therapy (prednisolone 60 mg daily). Failure to respond is an indication for orbital irradiation or surgical decompression. Orbital irradiation is administered by a linear accelerator over 10 fractions to a total dose of 2000 cGy. Over 80% of patients respond to irradiation. Alternatively orbital decompression may be achieved by either the transfrontal or transantral routes (Fig. 1.9). The transantral route is preferred because it is equally effective as the more extensive transfrontal operation but avoids a frontal craniotomy. About one-third of patients will develop diplopia after a transantral decompression so that an additional operation is required to correct it.

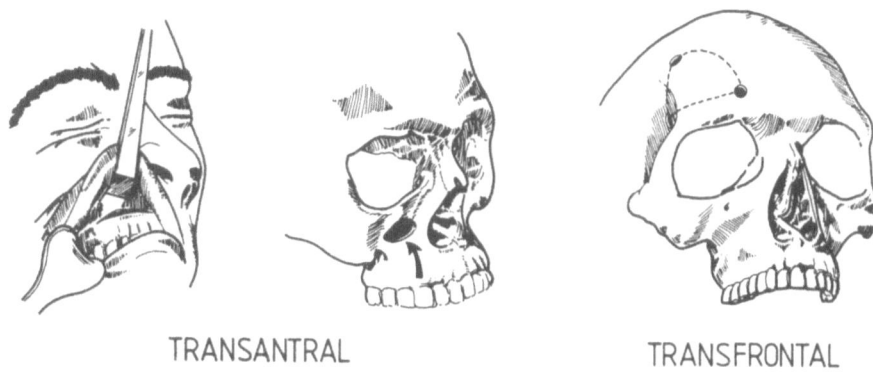

TRANSANTRAL   TRANSFRONTAL

Fig. 1.9. Transantral and transfrontal approaches to an orbital decompression for progressive endocrine exophthalmos.

2. *Multinodular goitre* should be treated by destructive therapy. Surgery is the treatment of choice and radioiodine is reserved for those who are unfit for surgery. These goitres are resistant to radioiodine and larger doses than those used for Graves' disease are employed. Usually 1200 MBq of ^{131}I is given. There is a high relapse rate following radioiodine and further doses may have to be given.

3. *An autonomous thyroid adenoma* is surrounded by normal thyroid tissue that is functionally suppressed and it was hoped that administered radioiodine would be selectively taken up by the adenoma resulting in its destruction and allowing the surrounding tissue to recover. Unfortunately this does not happen in practice—the nodule often fails to resolve and up to 36% of patients may become hypothyroid. Surgical excision is the best method of achieving a cure and involves a hemithyroidectomy of the affected side.

4. *Silent lymphocytic thyroiditis and subacute thyroiditis* are best treated by β-adrenoceptor blockade during the hyperthyroid phase but a short course of corticosteroids may shorten the period of hyperthyroidism dramatically.

5. *TSH-secreting pituitary tumours* are best treated by transsphenoidal microsurgery (see Chapter 3). If excess TSH secretion cannot be controlled by this method, hyperthyroidism may be controlled by radioiodine therapy but external pituitary irradiation is also indicated to prevent expansion of the pituitary tumour.

6. *Pituitary resistance to the action of thyroid hormones* is best controlled by ablation of the thyroid with radioiodine and subsequent replacement with L-thyroxine. Monitoring of the anterior pituitary with computerised tomography is necessary as subsequent thyrotroph hyperplasia may lead to expansion within the pituitary fossa. Combined pituitary and peripheral resistance requires treatment with L-thyroxine to suppress goitre formation and to treat underlying tissue hypothyroidism. However, the doses required to achieve

this will of necessity be high with great problems in assessing adequate replacement.

Euthyroid Goitres and Thyroid Cancer

These patients are euthyroid and usually present with a mass in the neck. Twelve per cent of women in the United Kingdom have a visible goitre; a further 12% have a palpable goitre that is not visible. The figures for men are 0.9% and 4.5% respectively.

Diagnosis

1. *Diffuse (simple) goitres* are commonly seen in iodine-deficient areas of the world and modest enlargement is often seen in young women during puberty and pregnancy. Eradication of iodine deficiency from some areas has dramatically reduced the prevalence of goitres. However, iodine deficiency is rarely the cause in the Western world and growth-receptor-stimulating antibodies may be responsible for goitre formation.

2. *Multinodular goitres* develop from diffuse (simple) goitres after several decades of autonomous stimulation. In the presence of an adequate iodine supply these euthyroid goitres may eventually evolve into hyperthyroid multinodular goitres.

3. *Single nodules* on palpation are classified by scintigraphy as "hot" or "cold". If the nodule is "hot" it is either a functioning adenoma or one nodule within a multinodular goitre. Although plasma thyroid hormones may be within the normal reference range, plasma TSH levels can be suppressed indicating autonomous function. Ten per cent of "cold" nodules and rarely "hot nodules" are thyroid cancers.

Traditionally all "cold" nodules are submitted to neck exploration but this means operating on 90% of patients with benign nodules to diagnose the 10% with malignancy. However, in many centres the introduction of fine-needle aspiration cytology is changing clinical practice (Fig. 1.10).

Aspiration is accomplished using a 10 ml disposable syringe and a 21-gauge 1.5 inch (green) disposable needle. The needle is inserted into the nodule and three passes made to obtain a representative sample. The plunger should be lightly retracted when in the target tissue and gently released as soon as a drop of blood is seen in the syringe tip. With the needle still in the target the syringe is disconnected and the needle is then withdrawn. The syringe is filled with air, the needle is reattached and the aspirate is then expelled on to a slide and smeared like a conventional blood film, air-dried or fixed in alcohol. The value of this method depends on obtaining a representative sample and having an expert cytologist to interpret it (Fig. 1.11). In good hands 93% of

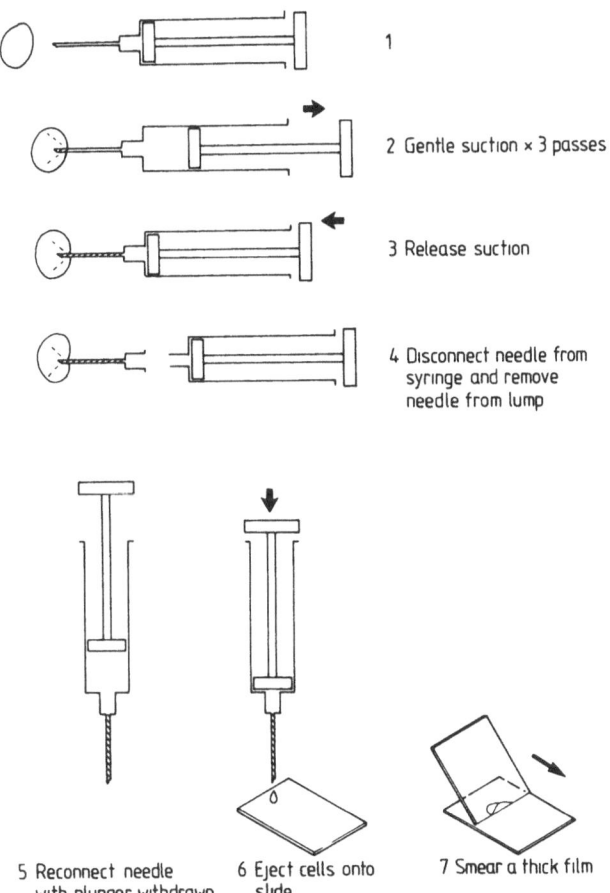

1

2 Gentle suction × 3 passes

3 Release suction

4 Disconnect needle from
  syringe and remove
  needle from lump

5 Reconnect needle   6 Eject cells onto   7 Smear a thick film
  with plunger withdrawn   slide

Fig. 1.10. Technique of aspiration cytology.

malignant tumours are correctly diagnosed with a false-negative rate of 7% and false-positive rate of less than 2%. Probable malignancies and doubtful cases should be submitted to surgery but this technique can reassure patient and physician that an operation can be avoided in many certain benign cases.

Thyroid cancer is uncommon with an annual incidence of approximately 5 per 100 000, encompassing a group of widely differing tumours ranging from slow-growing well-differentiated neoplasms with an excellent prognosis to anaplastic thyroid cancers that have a dismal outcome. Women are affected more than men. Fifty-five per cent of thyroid cancers are papillary carcinomas with a peak incidence in the third and fourth decades, 15% are follicular, 10% are anaplastic tumours developing in older patients in their sixth and seventh decades, 10% are lymphomas and 10% are medullary thyroid cancers.

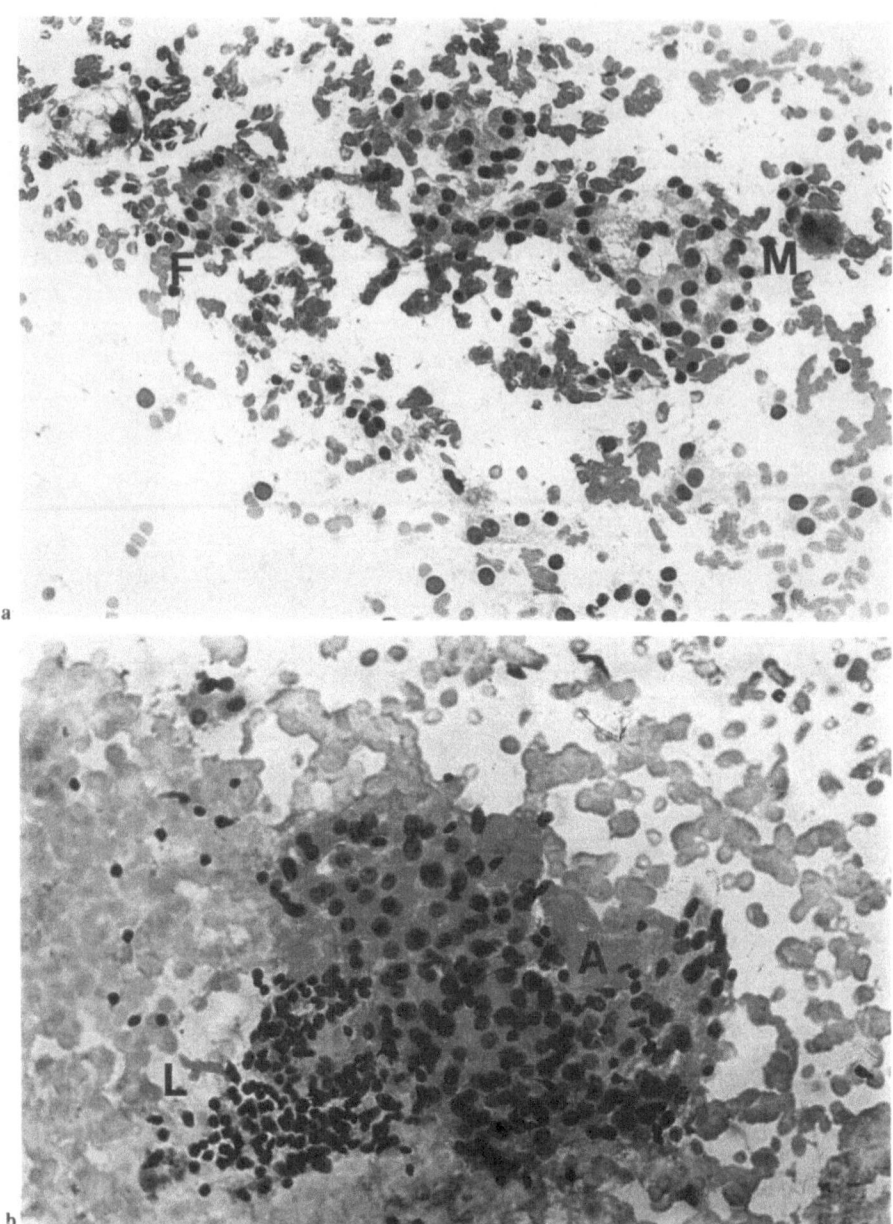

Fig. 1.11. Aspiration cytology demonstrating **a** a multinodular goitre with normal follicular cells (*F*) and an iron-laden macrophage (*M*), **b** Hashimoto's thyroiditis with transformed follicular cells (*A*, Ashkenazy cells).

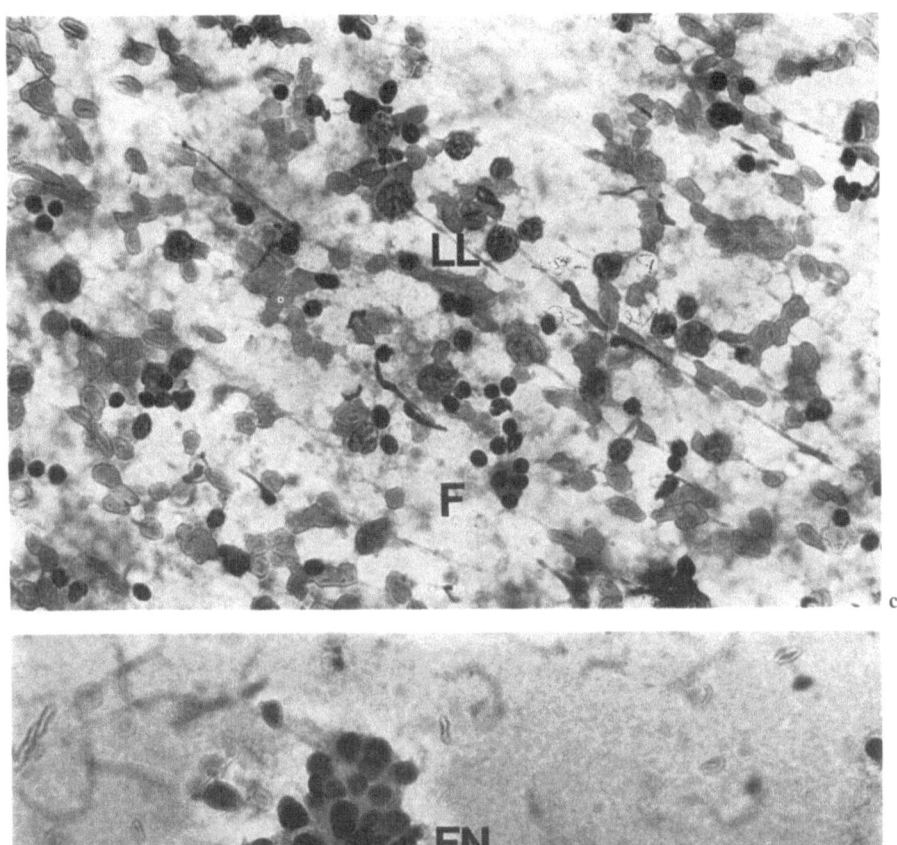

Fig. 1.11. (*continued*) **c** a lymphoma with normal follicular cells (*F*) and large lymphoid cells (*LL*) and **d** a follicular neoplasm with abnormal follicular cells (*FN*). (Courtesy Dr M McIntyre, Department of Pathology, Western General Hospital, Edinburgh.)

Medullary thyroid cancer is a tumour arising from the calcitonin-secreting parafollicular cells of the thyroid. It may arise sporadically or as part of a familial syndrome in association with multiple endocrine neoplasia (MEN) types 2 and 3.

Treatment

Diffuse (simple) multinodular goitres often do not require treatment but the patient should be assessed clinically, radiologically (plain X-ray of thoracic inlet) and with thyroid scintigraphy. Surgery is desirable for cosmetic reasons, where there is progressive enlargement or if signs of tracheal compression are present. These goitres do not usually shrink in response to the administration of L-thyroxine.

Single "hot" nodules should be followed up and appropriate therapy instituted if clinical or biochemical features of hyperthyroidism manifest themselves.

Thyroid cancer is treated according to the type of tumour. Sex and the age at diagnosis affect prognosis.

1. *Papillary cancers* present with a mass in the neck in 75% of cases and 33% have lymph node involvement at presentation. It is the size of the tumour that determines prognosis and tumours less than 15 mm in diameter appear to have no demonstrable mortality. Larger, more invasive tumours are more likely to cause death but even so 80%–90% of patients will survive several decades. In contrast, follicular cancers rarely spread to regional nodes but bone metastases occur early. The 10- and 20-year survival figures for follicular cancer are 34% and 10% respectively and angio-invasion on histology heralds a poorer prognosis.

The principles of therapy for these well-differentiated tumours are similar although follicular is less responsive than papillary cancer to radioiodine. Whilst it is possible to treat small papillary cancers by hemithyroidectomy and L-thyroxine suppression, thyroid ablation is the mainstay of treatment to eradicate multifocal disease and to make monitoring of metastases possible by ^{131}I whole body profile measurements and estimation of serum thyroglobulin. A near total thyroidectomy should be performed without being radical enough to increase the morbidity of the operation. Any residual tissue is destroyed by an ablative dose of 3000 MBq ^{131}I.

Subsequent hypothyroidism should be treated with triiodothyronine 20 μg 8-hourly by mouth as this has a shorter half-life than L-thyroxine. This is preferable because it is only necessary to stop the drug for 10 days prior to an ^{131}I whole body profile scan (Fig. 1.12) and estimation of serum thyroglobulin. This is performed 2 months after total ablation. Oral T_3 is restarted and serum thyroglobulin measurements are checked again with the concurrent estimation of plasma T_3 and TSH levels to ensure adequate TSH suppression (well-differentiated thyroid carcinomas are TSH-sensitive). If either the profile scan is positive or serum thyroglobulin elevated, a further ablation

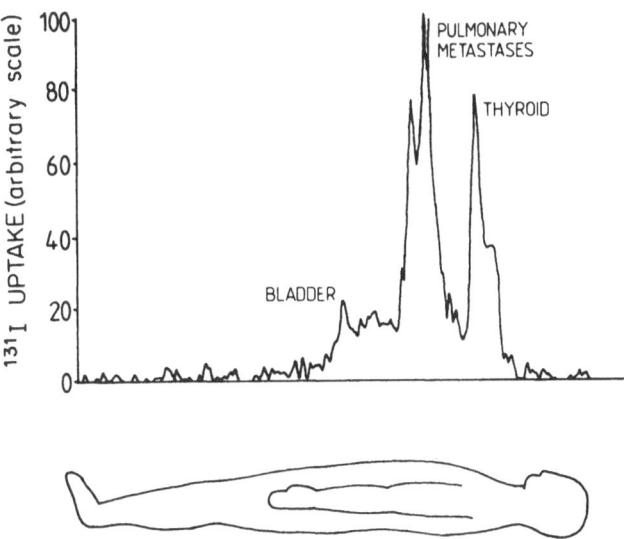

Fig. 1.12. ^{131}I whole body profile scan in a patient with metastatic follicular thyroid carcinoma. Whole body retention at 8 days, 1.5%; neck, 0.3%; thorax, 0.5%.

dose of ^{131}I is given. If these tests are negative the patient should be changed to a suppressive dose of L-thyroxine 200 µg daily. The neck should be examined annually and serum thyroglobulin monitored.

Unfortunately the corollary that an undetectable serum thyroglobulin means that the patient is free of metastases does not always hold true. Of those patients with negative profile scans, 2% will have detectable thyroglobulin on suppressive therapy rising to 16% on withdrawal of suppression. The former figure probably represents undetected residual cancer and the latter undetected normal thyroid tissue in the neck. Of those patients with scans indicating remnant in the neck, the respective figures are 24 and 61%, and 71 and 97% for those with scans indicating metastases. Clearly both of these methods are necessary to monitor the patient with thyroid cancer. Thus we would recommend that patients with well-differentiated thyroid cancer should have an annual examination and then be changed to triiodothyronine 20 µg 8-hourly for 6 weeks (to allow elimination of L-thyroxine) followed by triiodothyronine withdrawal for 10 days in order to repeat serum thyroglobulin estimations and a whole body profile scan. A positive scan or thyroglobulin estimation indicates metastases and further therapy (7000 mBq ^{131}I) should be given.

2. In contrast, *anaplastic thyroid cancer* is invariably fatal. The tumour is locally invasive and only palliative surgery is possible. Anaplastic cancers cause death in 90% of cases within 6 months, but the remaining 10% of patients may survive for up to 6 years or more. However, this may reflect the

difficulty in differentiating anaplastic tumours from lymphoma. Histological diagnosis can be improved in these patients by looking for lymphocyte surface markers. An alternative pragmatic policy is a trial of external irradiation — should a lymphoma be mistakenly diagnosed as an anaplastic tumour it will be recognised by its rapid response to radiotherapy.

3. Approximately 80% of *thyroid lymphomas* arise in glands previously involved by Hashimoto's or autoimmune thyroiditis. In the remainder, thyroid involvement is secondary to a systemic lymphoma. Malignant lymphomas arising within the thyroid are sensitive to external irradiation but chemotherapy is indicated for systemic involvement. Whilst local recurrence after radiotherapy is rare the 6-year survival following treatment is about 50%.

4. For *medullary thyroid cancer* the only effective treatment is surgery and 90% of patients without lymph node involvement will survive 10 years; this figure falls to 40% though with spread to regional nodes. Serum calcitonin levels can be used as a tumour marker and to screen relatives of those patients who have the familial form. These patients may be recognised by the presence of a multiple endocrine syndrome or the finding of C-cell hyperplasia in the normal thyroid tissue surrounding the carcinoma.

2 The Adrenal Gland

THE ADRENAL CORTEX

The steroids secreted by the adrenal cortex are principally glucocorticoid (cortisol), mineralocorticoid (aldosterone) and sex steroids (dehydroepiandrosterone, androstenedione, oestradiol and testosterone) (Fig. 2.1). The adrenal cortex is divided into three zones, with glucocorticoids and sex steroids being secreted by the zona reticularis and zona fasciculata, and mineralocorticoids by the zona glomerulosa. Cortisol secretion is regulated by the anterior pituitary secretion of ACTH (corticotrophin) but the major stimulus to the secretion of aldosterone is angiotensin II, formed by activation of the renin–angiotensin system. Sodium depletion not only stimulates the renin–angiotensin system but also enhances the responses of the zona glomerulosa to angiotensin II. Hyperkalaemia is another stimulus to aldosterone secretion. A factor other than ACTH has been suggested for the control of adrenal androgen production but evidence is far from convincing. In its turn ACTH is regulated by the hypothalamic secretion of corticotrophin-releasing factor (CRF).

The biological actions of glucocorticoid are concerned with intermediary metabolism, inflammation, immunity and wound healing. Glucocorticoids promote the conversion of protein to carbohydrate (gluconeogenesis) from amino acids in plasma and muscle and the storage of carbohydrate as liver glycogen from glucose. Thus, glucocorticoids increase protein breakdown with an increase in blood glucose but the subsequent rise in insulin secretion blocks the catabolic effects of corticosteroids by inhibiting lipolysis. Glucocorticoids increase body fat and enhance the lipolytic effect of catecholamines, but it is far from clear whether the changes in body fat reflect a direct effect or are due to stimulation of the appetite and enhanced caloric intake. Glucocorticoids are anti-inflammatory, inhibiting antibody production, reducing the number of anti-inflammatory cells mobilised to the area of inflammation, stabilising intracellular lysosomal membranes thus preventing the release of lysosomal enzymes and histamine from granulocytes, and inhibiting phospholipase A and the local production of prostaglandins. The suppression of these chemical mediators reduces capillary dilatation, permea-

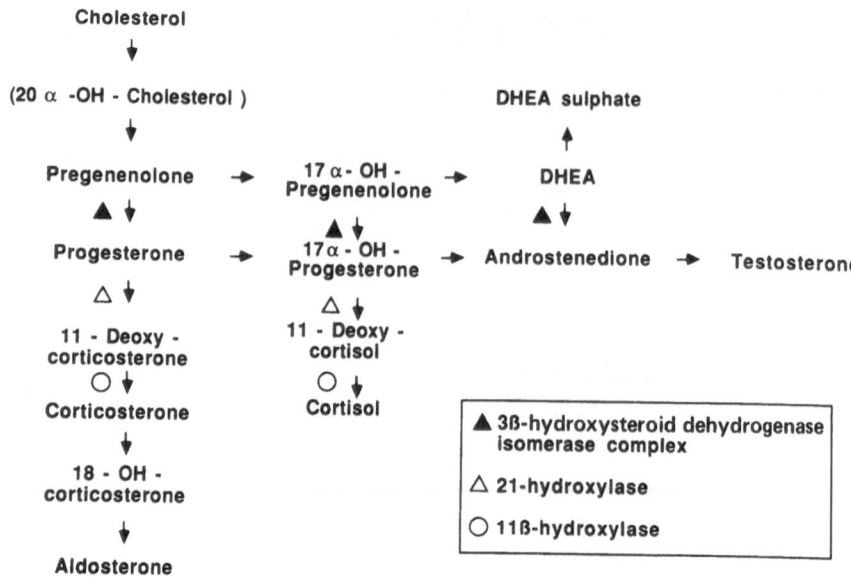

Fig. 2.1. The major pathways of synthesis of adrenal corticosteroids. (DHEA, dehydroepian-drosterone.)

bility and the subsequent volume of transudate. Glucocorticoids also interact with other endocrine systems, suppressing the anterior pituitary secretion of LH, GH and TSH but stimulating the enzyme PNMT which catalyses the conversion of noradrenaline to adrenaline as well as potentiating the β-adrenoceptor action of catecholamines. The adrenal cortex secretes approximately 20 mg of cortisol per day.

The secretion of corticosteroids follows a circadian pattern so that the plasma cortisol concentration is at its highest on wakening, falling throughout the day and reaching a minimum during the first hour of sleep. This circadian rhythm can be modified by sustained changes in sleep pattern and the pattern of light and dark; it is also altered by blindness. Both physiological and psychological stress, as well as hypoglycaemia, stimulate ACTH secretion overriding the circadian secretion of cortisol.

In the circulation, cortisol is bound to a specific protein, cortisol-binding globulin (CBG), as well as albumin and it is the free hormone that exerts biological activity. Since only free cortisol is filtered by the kidney, the 24-hour excretion of urinary cortisol is used as an index of free cortisol secretion. The estimated half-life of endogenous cortisol is approximately 60 minutes but this increases with the administration of pharmacological doses of cortisol. The rates of secretion and clearance are increased in hyperthyroidism and decreased in hypothyroidism. The plasma clearance rate is decreased in liver and renal diseases since these organs are the major sites of metabolism and excretion. The liver inactivates cortisol by reducing it to tetrahydrocortisol with the enzyme 3β-OH-steroid dehydrogenase, by converting it to cortisone with enzyme 11ß-OH-steroid dehydrogenase and subsequently forming tetrahydrocortisone, by hydroxylation to the more water-soluble 6β-hydroxycortisol, by side-chain cleavage and by conjugation with glucuronide and sulphate. The kidney filters free cortisol but approximately 90% of this is reabsorbed in the distal tubules whereas 6β-hydroxycortisol is readily excreted and conjugated steroids are filtered without reabsorption.

The major action of mineralocorticoids is to enhance the renal tubular reabsorption of sodium and the excretion of potassium by stimulating Na–K-ATPase. Aldosterone also acts on electrolyte transport in the gut and salivary glands. The influence of aldosterone on sodium retention, and hence plasma and extracellular fluid volume, plays an important role in the maintenance of normal blood pressure and cardiac output. Aldosterone secretion is stimulated by angiotensin II which is generated from angiotensin by the action of angiotensin-converting enzyme (ACE). This in turn is produced from angiotensinogen by the action of the enzyme renin. Renin is released from the juxtaglomerular apparatus of the kidney in response to a decrease in renal artery pressure. Thus plasma renin and aldosterone concentrations rise in response to assuming the erect posture, obscuring the normal ACTH-mediated circadian variation of aldosterone secretion which parallels that of cortisol (Fig. 2.2). The adrenal cortex secretes 0.19 mg of aldosterone per day which is metabolised in a similar fashion to cortisol to tetrahydro-aldosterone.

The physiologically potent adrenal androgen is testosterone, but this is only secreted in small amounts by the adrenal. The adrenal corticosteroids androstenedione, DHA and DHA-sulphate are weak androgens but can be converted in peripheral tissues to testosterone. Adrenal androgens are present in the blood in high concentrations following birth but become suppressed during infancy and childhood. However, as adolescence approaches the secretion of adrenal androgens increases (adrenarche). The mechanism of the adrenarche is unknown, but is independent of gonadotrophins and is responsible for the appearance of pubic and axillary hair in young girls and to a lesser extent in young boys. The adrenarche (occurring at age 6–7 in males and age 8–9 in females) usually precedes the gonadarche (occurring at age 12–14 in males and age 10–12 in females).

Adrenocortical Failure

Diagnosis

Hypocortisolaemia with Raised Plasma ACTH Levels

Primary adrenocortical failure (Addison's disease) is rare and is diagnosed on the basis of clinical features and the failure of the plasma cortisol to respond

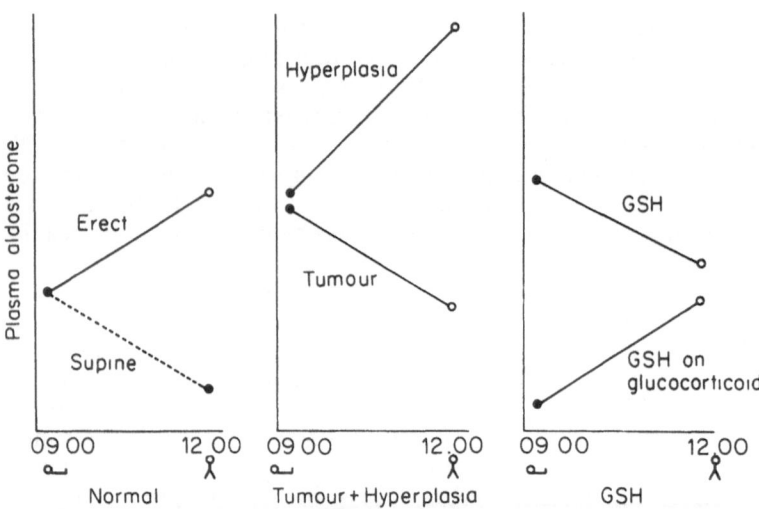

Fig. 2.2. Postural responses of plasma aldosterone concentrations. In normal individuals plasma aldosterone concentrations follow the normal cortisol and ACTH circadian rhythm providing the individual remains recumbent (●---●) but rise on standing (●—○) when the renin –angiotensin system is activated. Patients with an aldosterone-secreting adrenocortical tumour have plasma aldosterone concentrations that fail to respond to posture and follow the cortisol circadian rhythm. Patients with bilateral hyperplasia achieve an exaggerated response to posture with the exception of a rare subgroup (GSH) that behaves in a similar manner to a tumour but corrects to normal with the administration of suppressive doses of glucocorticoid.

to pharmacological doses of ACTH (250 μg tetracosactrin). Estimation of plasma ACTH with concomitant cortisol levels is used to confirm the diagnosis of primary adrenocortical failure and to differentiate it from secondary causes. However, no time should be wasted by delaying treatment of the patient until the result of the plasma ACTH estimation becomes available.

There are two major causes:

1. Autoimmune adrenalitis is the main cause of Addison's disease with an incidence of 27 per million.
2. Tuberculous Addison's disease has an incidence of 12 per million but is declining.

Other causes include metastatic cancer, sarcoidosis, septicaemia, drugs (aminoglutethimide, trilostane and etomidate), congenital adrenal hyperplasia and surgery.

Hypocortisolaemia with Low Plasma ACTH Levels

The causes of secondary adrenocortical insufficiency include pituitary or hypothalamic disease and suppression of the hypothalamic–pituitary–adrenal

(HPA) axis following the chronic administration and subsequent withdrawal of pharmacological doses of glucocorticoids. Suppression is achieved by daily doses of glucocorticoid in excess of 30 mg for hydrocortisone, 7.5 mg for prednisolone and 1 mg for dexamethasone. Glucocorticoid administered at night is more likely to cause suppression of the HPA axis than the same dose given in the morning. In secondary adrenal failure there is no significant loss of mineralocorticoid secretion as the adrenal cortex still remains responsive to the renin–angiotensin system.

Treatment

Acute adrenal insufficiency presents as an emergency with symptoms and signs resulting from salt and water depletion. Assessment should include estimation of pulse, supine blood pressure and, if this is normal, erect blood pressure to determine any degree of postural hypotension. Treatment is aimed at restoring a normal circulating blood volume with intravenous physiological saline (150 mmol/l). The amount of fluid replacement should be guided by the patient's condition and in particular pulse rate and erect and supine blood pressure. The blood sugar should also be measured and hypoglycaemia corrected with the administration of intravenous dextrosaline. Intravenous hydrocortisone 100 mg is administered as a bolus every 8 hours reducing to physiological doses when the patient has clinically recovered.

Chronic adrenal insufficiency is treated with physiological doses of glucocorticoid. Hydrocortisone (cortisol) is employed for glucocorticoid replacement in a dose of 20 mg by mouth before breakfast (food delays absorption) and 10 mg 8 hours later. Adequacy of cortisol replacement can then be ascertained by cortisol–ACTH day curves (Fig. 2.3). Mineralocorticoid is replaced by the oral administration of fludrocortisone 0.05–0.3 mg once daily. The dose is titrated by measurement of blood pressure, plasma electrolytes and plasma renin activity. Patients should be advised to double the dose of glucocorticoid in cases of acute stress such as a febrile illness or accident. They should also be encouraged to carry a card identifying that they are on corticosteroid replacement or, preferably, an identity bracelet. These can be obtained from Medicalert Foundation, 11/13 Clifton Terrace, London N4 3JP (tel. 01 263 8597). Patients with adrenal insufficiency undergoing acute surgery should be given an increased dose of steroid. For minor surgery 100 mg of intramuscular hydrocortisone is given with the premedication. For major operations this should be followed by 100 mg intramuscularly 8-hourly during day 1, reducing to 50 mg intramuscularly 8-hourly during day 2, and, provided the patient is unstressed and taking fluids by mouth, normal oral replacement can be recommenced on the 3rd postoperative day. Acute investigative procedures such as an angiogram can be safely covered by a single 100 mg dose of hydrocortisone either by mouth or intramuscularly if the patient is fasting.

Anticonvulsant drugs such as phenytoin, phenobarbitone and primidone as well as the antibiotic rifampicin increase the metabolism of glucocorticoids

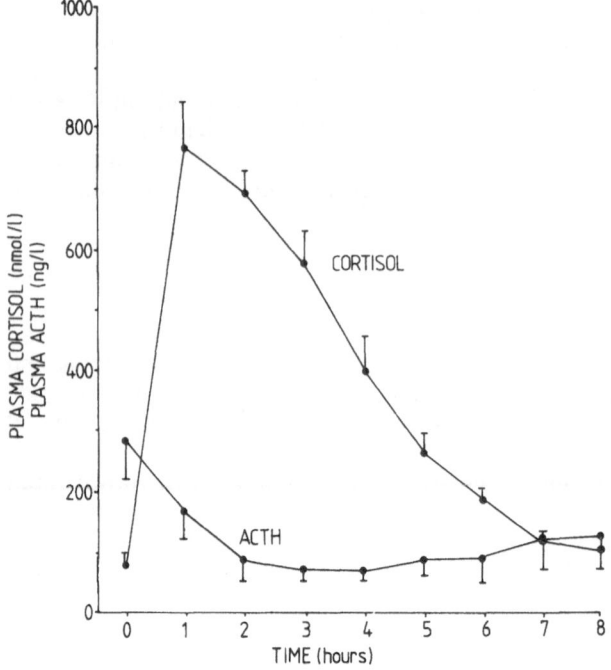

Fig. 2.3. Plasma cortisol and ACTH levels following the oral administration of hydrocortisone 20 mg in 12 patients with primary adrenal failure.

with a reduction of the therapeutic effect—larger doses of glucocorticoid may then be needed.

Glucocorticoid Excess

Diagnosis

Cushing's syndrome results from either the administration of supraphysiological amounts of glucocorticoid or ACTH, or from the sustained and inappropriate elevation of free plasma cortisol. The latter may be ACTH-dependent (either from the pituitary or an ectopic source) or ACTH-independent (adrenal adenoma or carcinoma). The specificity of the cortisol assay should be borne in mind when interpreting results. Cortisol has traditionally been estimated by a fluorometric method, and concomitant administration of drugs such as spironolactone may give falsely high results. Most laboratories now measure cortisol by specific radioimmunoassays but even these can mislead the unwary. Prednisolone cross-reacts with most anticortisol antibodies and will register as cortisol in the plasma assay. However, prednisolone does not interfere in the fluorometric assay and dexamethasone does not interfere significantly with either method. Patients are screened for investigation, selecting those in whom the plasma cortisol at 09.00 hours remains above 180 nmol/l after the administration of dexamethasone 2 mg at 23.00 hours the previous night. Investigation of a suspected patient is in two steps.

Firstly, demonstration of inappropriate hypercortisolaemia:

1. Loss of circadian rhythm of plasma cortisol with elevated levels at midnight.

2. Elevated 24-hour urinary free cortisol excretion (or cortisol/creatinine ratio on an early morning specimen).

3. Lack of suppressibility of 09.00 hour plasma cortisol levels following the oral administration of dexamethasone 0.5 mg 6-hourly for 2 days (low dose).

4. Absent or blunted plasma cortisol response to insulin-induced hypoglycaemia.

Secondly, demonstration of the cause of the syndrome:

1. Plasma ACTH levels at 09.00 hours.

2. Plasma cortisol response to the oral administration of dexamethasone 2 mg 6-hourly for 2 days (high dose).

3. Plasma 11-deoxycortisol response to the oral administration of metyrapone (an 11β-hydroxylase inhibitor which blocks the synthesis of cortisol, increasing ACTH secretion and stimulating the formation of precursors such as 11-deoxycortisol) in a dose of 750 mg 4-hourly for 24 hours.

Hypercortisolaemia with Detectable Plasma ACTH Levels

Approximately 80% of cases of Cushing's syndrome are pituitary in origin (Cushing's disease) and 10% are due to ectopic hormone production. Alcohol-induced Cushing's syndrome is now well recognised as a reversible cause of glucocorticoid excess.

A pituitary cause is indicated by detectable plasma ACTH levels, suppression of plasma cortisol during high-dose dexamethasone administration and plasma 11-deoxycortisol levels in excess of 1000 nmol/l following metyrapone. Further investigations should include plain skull radiography and computerised tomography of the pituitary.

An ectopic source of ACTH is suggested when plasma ACTH is detectable, plasma 11-deoxycortisol levels are less than 1000 nmol/l following metyrapone and plasma cortisol levels fail to suppress with high-dose dexamethasone. In addition, in ectopic cases there is usually no plasma ACTH response to the intravenous administration of CRF, whereas in cases due to a corticotrophinoma there is a fourfold increment. Another very important pointer to the diagnosis of ectopic ACTH syndrome is the presence of a hypokalaemic alkalosis. Whole body computerised tomography and selective venous sampling (if possible with bilateral blood sampling from the inferior petrosal sinus) should be performed as necessary and blood taken for assessment of other tumour markers.

The diagnosis of alcohol-induced Cushing's syndrome should be suspected if there are obvious features of chronic alcoholism. Estimation of plasma ACTH levels in these patients has been variable. Biochemical features of hypercortisolaemia disappear over a few days of alcohol withdrawal.

Hypercortisolaemia with Undetectable Plasma ACTH Levels

Primary adrenal tumours account for approximately 10% of cases of Cushing's syndrome. In primary adrenal causes, plasma ACTH levels are undetectable, plasma 11-deoxycortisol response to metyrapone is blunted and there is usually no plasma cortisol response to dexamethasone. The abnormal adrenal is localised by computerised tomography and ^{75}Se-cholesterol adrenal scintigraphy which will confirm that the contralateral adrenal is suppressed. Adrenal carcinomas may show no uptake of labelled cholesterol.

Treatment

Oral metyrapone may be given in a dose of 250 mg 6-hourly to prepare patients for surgery and the dose titrated to the plasma cortisol profile throughout the day to maintain plasma cortisol levels between 330 and 400 nmol/l. However, treatment of the various causes of Cushing's syndrome is surgical where possible:

1. Corticotrophinoma: the surgical approach to treatment is discussed under the section on the pituitary.
2. Successful surgical removal of an ectopic tumour secreting ectopic ACTH depends on its nature and site.
3. Primary adrenal tumours are best removed surgically by a loin incision on the affected side, morbidity being less than with a "suitcase" incision of the anterior abdominal wall. Following unilateral adrenal surgery there is a period of adrenocortical insufficiency whilst the ACTH-secreting cells of the pituitary and the suppressed contralateral adrenal recover. This may last for 6 months to 2 years and patients are best treated with dexamethasone 0.5 mg by mouth in the morning as this is less suppressive than an evening dose, less than physiological replacement and does not interfere in the assay for plasma cortisol which should be used to monitor recovery. Irresectable adrenal carcinomas may be treated with the adrenolytic drug o,p'-DDD but this is a palliative manoeuvre.

Mineralocorticoid Excess

Diagnosis

Hyperaldosteronism with Suppressed Plasma Renin Levels

Primary hyperaldosteronism is an uncommon cause of hypertension accounting for less than 1% of unselected hypertensives. However, it should always be considered in patients in whom an elevated blood pressure is associated with hypernatraemia and hypokalaemic alkalosis. The pathogenesis of this condition is due to an adrenocortical adenoma or idiopathic hyperplasia. These two conditions are distinguished by the plasma aldosterone response to posture (Fig. 2.2), the estimation of plasma 18-hydroxycortisol [very high in adenomas or GSH (see below); minimally elevated in common idiopathic hyperplasia], computerised tomography and adrenal scintigraphy. There is a rare subgroup of patients with idiopathic hyperplasia in which plasma aldosterone responses are similar to those of a tumour (glucocorticoid-suppressible hyperaldosteronism, GSH). In this condition hyperaldosteronism can be cured by suppression of the HPA axis with the oral administration of glucocorticoid, reducing plasma aldosterone to normal levels which respond to posture. Patients in whom there is a postural fall in aldosterone should be given dexamethasone 0.5 mg 8-hourly for 14 days after which blood pressure and plasma aldosterone concentrations are measured to detect those who may have GSH. Scintigraphy is successful in diagnosing the cause of primary hyperaldosteronism in 75% of cases but may be adversely affected by previous long-term treatment with spironolactone. In some patients, particularly those with small tumours, adrenal vein catheterisation with measurement of aldosterone and cortisol levels may be necessary to localise the lesion.

Hyperaldosteronism with Raised Plasma Renin Levels

Secondary hyperaldosteronism occurs in four main groups of conditions:

1. When there is extrarenal sodium loss, such as in haemorrhage or gastrointestinal fluid loss, and aldosterone secretion is a physiological response to hypovolaemia and reduces renal sodium loss.

2. When there is oedema, such as in cardiac failure, liver failure and nephrotic syndrome, and aldosterone secretion results from a contracted plasma volume. This is often exacerbated by diuretic therapy.

3. When renin secretion is either due to renal ischaemia, renal artery stenosis, accelerated phase hypertension or a renin-secreting tumour.

4. When impaired reabsorption of salt is a primary renal abnormality, such as in salt-losing nephritis, diuretic abuse and Bartter's syndrome, or where the effect of aldosterone on the kidney is impaired (such as in pregnancy).

Treatment

Aldosterone-secreting tumours are almost always benign and should be treated by unilateral adrenalectomy. After removal of the adenoma, aldosterone (but not cortisol) secretion is suppressed in the contralateral adrenal so that postoperative hyperkalaemia may be a problem until recovery ensues. This may be avoided by preoperative preparation with spironolactone, a competitive antagonist of aldosterone. A daily dose of 400 mg is given by mouth for 6 weeks, rapidly correcting the hypertension and hypokalaemia. Unfortunately some 40% of patients remain hypertensive following surgery when followed for up to 10 years. If surgery is contraindicated or refused, long-term medical treatment is recommended with spironolactone. Unfortunately this drug can act as an antiandrogen and about 20% of men develop gynaecomastia and impotence. An alternative drug is amiloride, which is an inhibitor of renal tubular ionic transport and is usually given in doses of up to 40 mg daily.

In idiopathic hyperplasia the blood pressure does not usually respond to spironolactone. Recent studies have shown that in this condition the zona glomerulosa is abnormally sensitive to angiotensin II and the condition can be treated by the oral administration of angiotensin-converting enzyme inhibitor such as captopril in a dose of 12.5–25 mg 8-hourly. GSH usually responds to the administration of glucocorticoid given in a manner to suppress the HPA axis (a reversed circadian pattern of glucocorticoid, prednisolone 2.5 mg in the morning and dexamethasone 0.5 mg before going to bed). Surgery is contraindicated for patients with idiopathic hyperplasia.

Secondary hyperaldosteronism is treated by attention to the underlying condition. Heart failure should be treated by conventional means including the administration of a loop-acting diuretic such as frusemide. In addition this condition can be treated by the oral administration of an angiotensin-converting enzyme inhibitor such as captopril in a dose of 6.25–25 mg 8-hourly. Captopril should not be used in the treatment of bilateral renal artery stenosis because renal failure may be precipitated. Renal artery stenosis is now being treated by transluminal angioplasty in many centres.

Adrenocortical Androgen Excess

Adrenal androgen overproduction occurs in the commonest type of congenital adrenal hyperplasia (CAH) due to 21-hydroxylase deficiency. This is an autosomal recessive disorder of cortisol biosynthesis with subsequent excess ACTH secretion. Increased secretion of ACTH results in increased secretion of those steroid precursors in the pathway prior to the defect in cortisol production and hence adrenal hyperplasia. Symptoms result from glucocorticoid insufficiency, mineralocorticoid insufficiency and adrenal androgen overproduction. Deficiency of 21-hydroxylase enzyme accounts for 90% of cases of CAH. Its incidence is approximately 1 in 13 000 live births. Virilisation is the cardinal clinical feature, resulting in ambiguous genitalia of the newborn female infant and precocious puberty in the male. Symptoms of salt loss occur in the 2nd week of life in 50% of the cases, characterised by vomiting, dehydration, circulatory collapse, hyponatraemia and hyperkalaemia.

Diagnosis

It is essential to confirm the clinical diagnosis with appropriate biochemical tests as soon as possible to start early glucocorticoid and if necessary

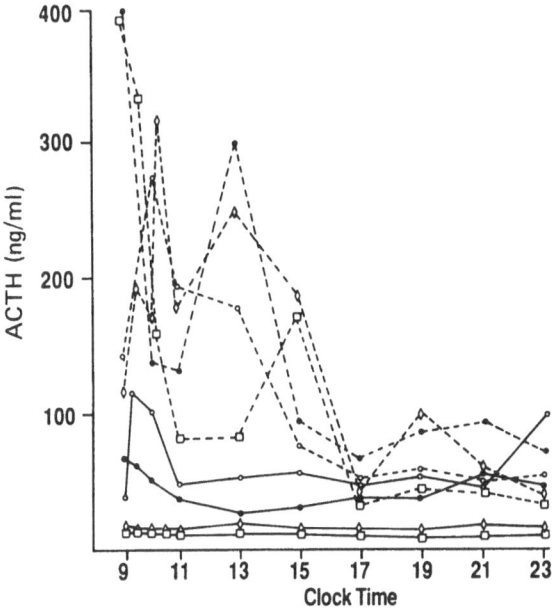

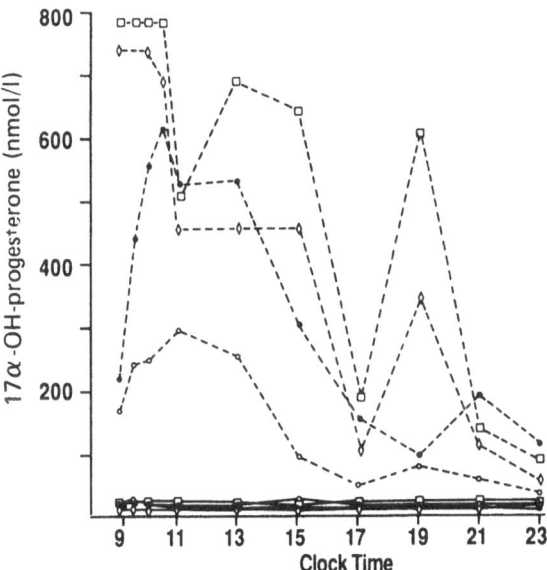

Fig. 2.4. Plasma ACTH and 17α-OH-progesterone levels in four patients with congenital hyperplasia before (– – –) and after (——) treatment with oral dexamethasone on retiring and prednisolone 2.5 mg on waking.

mineralocorticoid replacement. Serum levels of 17α-OH-progesterone are markedly elevated in untreated 21-hydroxylase deficiency (in excess of 200 nmol/l). However, plasma 17α-OH-progesterone levels can be elevated within hours of birth in normal infants and the collection of blood should be delayed until the 2nd day of life when plasma levels are less than 6 nmol/l.

Treatment

Acute salt-losing crisis is immediately treated by the intravenous administration of physiological saline with 5% dextrose and hydrocortisone.

The aim of long-term therapy in CAH is to provide sufficient glucocorticoid replacement therapy to suppress excess adrenal androgen secretion to allow normal growth during childhood, normal pubertal development and adult reproductive potential. Often hydrocortisone in doses of 10–20 mg/m^2/day in three divided doses is recommended but small doses of longer acting synthetic glucocorticoids given at night may provide better control of precursor secretion. It is easier to suppress the HPA axis with the administration of the major dose of glucocorticoid at night. Excessive glucocorticoid must be avoided as this inhibits both the release of growth hormone and its biological effects. In older children and adults prednisolone 2.5 mg orally is given on waking and dexamethasone 0.5 mg on retiring at night (Fig. 2.4). This regimen achieves adequate suppression of plasma ACTH, cortisol and 17α-OH-progesterone concentrations. In females the most discriminating monitor of successful therapy is the development of normal menstruation and fertility. The need for such strict control in postpubertal males is debatable. Mineralocorticoid therapy is assessed by blood pressure, plasma electrolytes and plasma renin levels.

THE ADRENAL MEDULLA

The adrenal medulla is functionally a giant presynaptic sympathetic nerve ending capable of synthesising noradrenaline and adrenaline. Phenylethanolamine N-methyltransferase (PNMT), the enzyme that converts noradrenaline to adrenaline, is only found in the adrenal gland so that excessive adrenaline secretion is suggestive of an adrenal medullary source of catecholamines. The most routinely measured urinary metabolites are vanillylmandelic acid (VMA), total metadrenaline and normetadrenaline.

Catecholamine Excess

Phaeochromocytomas are rare tumours of the adrenal medulla and sympathetic nervous system accounting for only 0.5% of cases of hypertension. These tumours may be sporadic or familial. Approximately 90% of the sporadic cases have their origin in the adrenal gland (81% being unilateral and 9% bilateral), 6% are extra-adrenal and in 4% of cases multiple. Phaeochromocytomas are reported in association with familial syndromes—MEN (multiple endocrine neoplasia) type 2, MEN type 3, multiple neurofibromatosis (Von Recklinghausen's disease) and diseases of the neuroectoderm (von Hippel–Lindau disease, tuberous sclerosis and cerebellar haemangioma). Approximately 82% of familial phaeochromocytomas are located within the adrenal gland (35% being unilateral and 47% bilateral), 8% extra-adrenal and 10% multiple. In MEN syndromes associated with phaeochromocytoma, the tumours are invariably bilateral. Less than 10% of phaeochromocytomas are malignant, the diagnosis being made on the basis of biological behaviour rather than histology. Clinical manifestations of these tumours result from the excessive release of catecholamines into the circulation. Although the majority of patients with phaeochromocytomas have symptoms most of the time, fluctuations in severity are perceived as paroxysms in 50%. Long-term complications include cerebrovascular accidents, retinopathy, nephropathy, psychiatric disturbance, glucose intolerance, myocardial infarction and heart failure. In addition, catecholamines may produce a cardiomyopathy.

Diagnosis

Of the three biochemical tests used to establish the diagnosis of phaeochromocytoma, estimation of urinary VMA is the least helpful, being elevated in only 50% of phaeochromocytomas with many false-positives. Urinary total metadrenaline and normetadrenaline are elevated in 80% of cases and reflect plasma adrenaline and noradrenaline levels respectively. However, plasma catecholamines are elevated in 90%–95% of cases, ranging from 2 to 30 times normal. If plasma catecholamines are equivocal, blood should be taken before and 10 minutes after the intravenous administration of pentolinium 2.5 mg. Pentolinium inhibits adrenaline and noradrenaline secretion from adrenergic nerve endings in normal individuals but will fail to suppress autonomous secretion by a functioning adrenal tumour. In normal individuals plasma adrenaline and noradrenaline levels suppress below 2 and 5 nmol/l respectively. A variety of other pharmacological tests have been employed in the diagnosis of phaeochromocytoma but are now obsolete because of lack of specificity and inherent dangers encountered with some of the agents used.

As soon as the diagnosis has been confirmed medical therapy should be instituted.

1. α-*Adrenoceptor blocking drugs* reduce blood pressure and ameliorate symptoms. Such treatment will allow expansion of the vascular bed and plasma volume but postural hypotension may be marked at the beginning of therapy until this is achieved. Persistent postural hypotension accompanied by evidence of a reduced plasma volume is occasionally an indication for plasma expansion. α-Adrenoceptor blockade is achieved by the administration of phenoxybenzamine, a non-competitive α-antagonist with a prolonged effect. Treatment is begun with doses of 20–40 mg daily and increased if necessary until adequate blood pressure control is achieved. Completely normal blood pressures are not always obtainable.

2. β-*Adrenoceptor blocking drugs* should be introduced after α-blockade to prevent catecholamine-induced arrhythmias. Propranolol is employed in a dose of 40–80 mg 8-hourly. β-Adrenoceptor blocking drugs should not be given alone because in the absence of α-blockade intense peripheral vasoconstriction may cause alarming rises in blood pressure. Labetalol, a mixed α- and β-adrenoreceptor blocking drug, is often recommended for the management of phaeochromocytomas. However it is predominantly a β-antagonist drug and therefore may elevate rather than reduce blood pressure (Fig. 2.5). It is essential that therapy is instituted prior to any invasive investigative procedure.

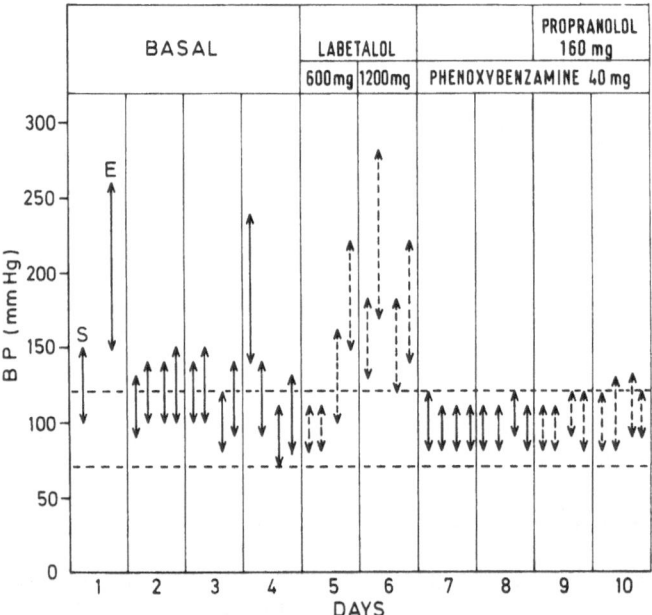

Fig. 2.5. Blood pressure estimations (E, erect; S, supine) in a patient with a phaeochromocytoma before and after oral treatment with labetalol, followed by subsequent treatment with a combination of oral phenoxybenzamine and propranolol (see text for details).

Localisation of the tumour is necessary to facilitate surgical removal. Methods of imaging currently employed are ultrasound, computerised tomography and more recently [131]I-*meta*-iodobenzylguanidine scintigraphy. Ultrasound is a readily available method of localising adrenal tumours but is poor at localising extra-adrenal sites. Computerised tomography will detect approximately 90%–100% of unilateral and bilateral adrenal tumours but only 60% of those that are extra-adrenal. Scintigraphy will yield very similar results but has the advantage over computerised tomography of being able to image the whole body and is therefore better at locating metastases. Whilst these methods can easily locate the larger tumours they may be unsuccessful with smaller ones. In these cases selective venous sampling is helpful with blood sample analysis for catecholamines. Arteriography is inherently dangerous.

Definitive treatment of phaeochromocytoma is surgical and despite preoperative preparation remains a hazardous procedure. The two major problems encountered are:

1. Acute elevations in blood pressure and arrhythmias with handling of the tumour. Sodium nitroprusside, a smooth muscle relaxant, is used to control intra-operative rises in blood pressure and arrhythmias are controlled by the intravenous administration of a β-blocker (Fig. 2.6).

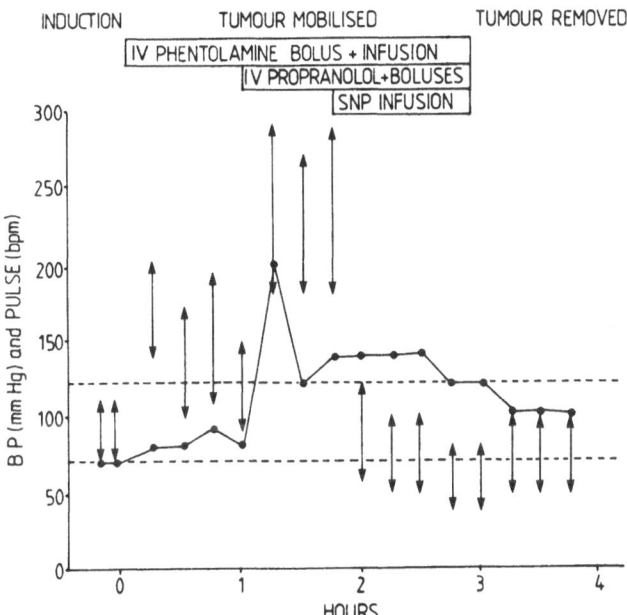

Fig. 2.6. Pulse rate and blood pressure estimations in a patient undergoing surgery for a phaeochromocytoma. SNP, sodium nitroprusside.

2. The precipitous fall in blood pressure following removal of the tumour is caused by a combination of plasma volume expansion and down-regulation of adrenergic receptors. Postoperative shock is treated with plasma expansion and if necessary infusion of noradrenaline but this will only delay recovery of adrenergic receptors.

3 The Ovary

After birth there is a prolonged period of gonadal inactivity that ends with the initiation of puberty. These changes result from suppression and withdrawal of suppression of the hypothalamic secretion of gonadotrophin releasing hormone (GnRH). In response to messages it receives from central and autonomic nervous systems the hypothalamus generates an intermittent pulse signal secreting a bolus of GnRH approximately every 90 minutes. With the onset of puberty, the pulsatile secretion of GnRH stimulates the anterior pituitary nocturnally to release luteinising hormone (LH) and to a lesser extent follicle-stimulating hormone (FSH). Under the influence of FSH a single follicle is selected and matured to produce an ovum. During this process the follicle enlarges as a result of an increase in the number of cells (theca interna and granulosa) and the ovum undergoes the later stages of meiosis prior to ovulation. The cells of the theca interna secrete androstenedione which is subsequently converted by the granulosa cells to oestradiol and oestrone. This results in a marked rise in blood oestrogen levels during the 5 days before ovulation. The rise in oestrogens exerts positive feedback at the level of the anterior pituitary resulting in a massive discharge of LH. It is this discharge of LH that causes rupture of the matured follicle and ovulation. Whilst oestrogens classically cause negative feedback inhibition of GnRH and gonadotrophin secretion, the mechanism of mid-cycle positive feedback is unclear. The mechanism probably involves increased sensitivity of the anterior pituitary to GnRH, as well as increased discharge of GnRH resulting from the changing levels of oestrogen secretion and progesterone secretion just before ovulation.

Following ovulation the follicle is transformed into the corpus luteum, the role of which is to secrete progesterone as well as oestrogen. The main target for these hormones is the uterus. During the first half of the menstrual cycle (proliferative phase) oestrogens stimulate glandular growth of the endometrium and induce the formation of progesterone receptors in preparation for the second half of the cycle (secretory phase) during which the endometrium is maintained by high levels of progesterone prior to implantation of an embryo. Thus the life of the endometrium depends on the short life-span of the corpus luteum unless implantation of an embryo occurs with secretion of human chorionic gonadotrophin (hCG) to maintain it. Menstruation occurs as progesterone levels fall, secretion by the

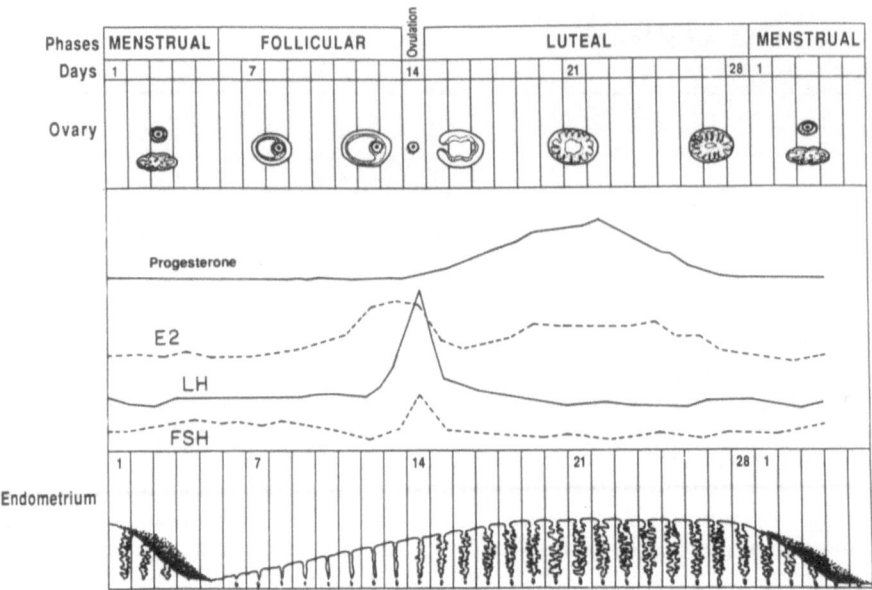

Fig. 3.1. The normal menstrual cycle. E₂, oestradiol; LH, luteinising hormone; FSH, follicle stimulating hormone.

endometrium diminishes, the spiral arteries contract and the surface layers die and are shed (Fig. 3.1).

Early in puberty many cycles occur without ovulation and cycles are often erratic until a more regular rhythm is established with an average cycle length of 25–30 days. The most obvious secondary sexual changes of female puberty are the development of breasts and the distribution of body fat. Oestrogens stimulate the growth of breast epithelium which in turn stimulates the local fat-cell growth that is responsible for most of the increase in breast volume. Progesterone also increases the volume of the oestrogen-primed breast whereas prolactin is only important in stimulating lactation.

Hypogonadism

Diagnosis

Hypogonadism with Raised Plasma Gonadotrophins

Primary gonadal failure usually presents with either a failure of normal pubertal development and primary amenorrhoea, or later in adult life with the symptoms of oestrogen deficiency (loss of libido, hot flushes and vaginal dryness) and secondary amenorrhoea. It can be confirmed by the finding of low plasma oestradiol and elevated plasma gonadotrophin concentrations. There are several causes:

1. Physiological ovarian failure occurs with the menopause when the supply of follicles that can be selected for ovulation becomes exhausted.

2. Gonadal dysgenesis and sex-chromosome abnormalities present with primary amenorrhoea and failure of development of secondary sex characteristics. There may be phenotypic features to suggest Turner's syndrome, such as webbing of the neck, low hairline, shield-shaped chest and increased carrying angle. Absent ovaries can be confirmed by ovarian ultrasound and any chromosome abnormality by peripheral leucocyte culture.

3. Autoimmune destruction of the ovaries can occur in female patients with autoimmune Addison's disease when the antibody directed against the adrenal cortex cross-reacts with steroid-secreting cells in the ovary.

4. Miscellaneous causes include pelvic irradiation and cancer chemotherapy.

Hypogonadism with Normal or Low Plasma Gonadotrophin Levels

Secondary ovarian failure can be the result of several causes and is diagnosed by the finding of low plasma gonadotrophins and low plasma oestrogens.

1. *Weight-related amenorrhoea* is a common condition. It is necessary for a female to reach a critical body weight before menstruation and ovulation occur. This is approximately 40 kg but obviously varies according to the individual's ideal body weight. The female is particularly susceptible to the disturbances of hypothalamic control of gonadotrophin secretion that occurs in anorexia nervosa and in athletes and ballet dancers. Ovarian ultrasound often reveals the presence of multicystic ovaries (cf. polycystic ovaries) in these patients.

2. *Isolated GnRH deficiency* occurs in Kallmann's syndrome and is usually associated with anosmia.

3. *Pituitary and para-pituitary lesions (including hyperprolactinaemia)* are discussed in Chapter 5.

4. *Delayed puberty.*

Treatment

Sex hormone replacement should be given to all women with primary ovarian failure until the time that they would be expected to have a normal menopause. It is established that oestrogens protect the skeleton against postmenopausal bone loss and improve symptoms of oestrogen deficiency. Oral ethinyloestradiol (10–20 µg daily) is the simplest to use and should be given from day 1 to day 21 of the menstrual cycle in combination with medroxyprogesterone acetate (5 mg daily) from day 14 to day 21 to prevent endometrial hyperplasia and the risk of endometrial carcinoma.

Treatment of secondary ovarian failure should naturally be directed at the underlying cause (treatment of hyperprolactinaemia is discussed in Chapter 5) but irreversible sex-steroid deficiency should be treated with hormone replacement therapy. If fertility is required, induction of ovulation may be attempted by the following pharmacological means:

1. *Anti-oestrogen* treatment with clomiphene citrate acting at the level of the hypothalamus increases the pulse frequency of GnRH secretion and potentiates the anterior pituitary LH response to GnRH. Provided oestrogen-mediated feedback is intact clomiphene is a useful agent in the induction of ovulation. An oral dose of 50–100 mg daily is usually given on days 1–5 of each menstrual cycle and the response may be monitored by estimation of the day 21 plasma progesterone concentration (a level in excess of 30 nmol/l is indicative of adequate ovulation). Treatment with clomiphene can make pregnancy possible in approximately 30% of women with anovulatory infertility but 10% of these pregnancies are multiple (usually twins), compared with a rate of 1.25% in normal pregnancies. Side-effects are few but patients may experience disturbances of peripheral vision particularly at dawn and dusk.

2. *Gonadotrophin therapy* is indicated for those patients with low plasma oestrogen concentrations as clomiphene is ineffective in its absence. Treatment with gonadotrophin involves two stages—induction of follicular maturation followed by induction of ovulation. Menotrophin (human menopausal gonadotrophin), containing both LH (75 units) and FSH (75 units) per ampoule, is administered daily in a dose of 1–2 ampoules per day by intramuscular injection until follicular development is adequate. This is usually achieved within 10 to 15 days but the patient's response must be carefully monitored with ovarian ultrasound and estimation of either plasma or urinary oestrogen concentrations. The aim of treatment is to achieve plasma oestradiol concentrations of between 1100 and 3000 pmol/l. Plasma oestrogen levels below this range indicate inadequate follicular development and levels in excess of this range indicate a risk of hyperstimulation if human chorionic gonadotrophin (hCG) is administered in the second phase of treatment. In its full-blown form the hyperstimuiation syndrome consists of massive ovarian enlargement, ascites and hydrothorax. Once appropriate plasma oestrogen levels have been achieved a single dose of hCG is given intramuscularly in a dose of 10 000 units to induce ovulation. The patient is recommended to have coitus on the day, as well as the day after, the hCG injection. Ovulation can be induced in almost all patients and a successful pregnancy can be expected in approximately 60%. Unfortunately the major drawback of this form of treatment is the risk of multiple pregnancy (mainly twin births) with a rate that varies between 10% and 40%. For this reason and because of expense, gonadotrophin therapy is being replaced in patients with residual gonado-trophin function by the administration of GnRH. Needless to say, treatment with gonadotrophins should only be undertaken in specialised centres with access to rapid oestrogen assays and ovarian ultrasound.

3. *Pulsatile GnRH therapy* is delivered by means of a portable pulsatile pump that mimics the natural secretion of GnRH. A dose of 10–20 μg is given subcutaneously every 90 minutes and treatment should be continued until a pregnancy is achieved or for a maximum of 6 months. Estimation of day 21 plasma progesterone concentrations and ovarian ultrasound may be used to monitor therapy but such surveillance is often unnecessary. Sixty per cent of patients with gonadotrophin insufficiency may be expected to conceive within three cycles of treatment. The plasma LH and FSH response to the intravenous administration of GnRH (GnRH test: see Chapter 5) does not seem to predict those patients who will respond to pulsatile GnRH therapy. The cumulative conception rate following pulsatile GnRH in those patients with multicystic ovaries (weight-related amenorrhoea) is 84% within three cycles of treatment but treatment is less successful in those patients with the polycystic ovarian syndrome (see later in this chapter) in whom the 3-month cumulative conception rate is only 35%. There is some evidence that this can be improved by giving intravenous rather than subcutaneous GnRH. Unlike gonadotrophin therapy, the risk of hyperstimulation is low with pulsatile GnRH and the multiple pregnancy rate is 3%, which approaches that of a normal pregnancy (1.25%).

Hypergonadism: Precocious Puberty

Diagnosis

Development of oestrogen-dependent secondary sex characteristics before the age of 9 years in females is usually abnormal. The abnormality may arise from a variety of causes:

1. Secretion of sex steroids in the absence of activation of gonadotrophin secretion is usually accompanied by an absence of ovulation. This can be due to either adrenal or ovarian tumours. Virilisation will occur if there is increased secretion of testosterone or other androgens.

2. Premature activation of the hypothalamic–pituitary axis (idiopathic precocious puberty) as in normal puberty leads to cyclical secretion of sex steroids, menstruation and ovulation. This is the commonest cause of precocious puberty in girls.

3. Other causes of premature gonadotrophin secretion include primary hypothyroidism, the McCune–Albright syndrome (polyostotic fibrous dysplasia, skin pigmentation and precocious puberty), neurofibromatosis and some types of hypothalamic disease. It is rarely associated with pineal tumours.

Treatment

Total surgical removal is the obvious treatment for adrenal or ovarian tumours where feasible. Idiopathic precocious puberty and syndromes involving premature gonadotrophin secretion are best managed by the chronic administration of long-acting GnRH analogues which cause "down-regulation" of anterior pituitary gonadotrophin receptors, regression of secondary sex characteristics and which stop acceleration of bone age. Buserelin may be given by the intra-nasal route in doses of 200 µg twice daily.

Hypergonadism: Hirsutism

Hirsutism in women may be defined as excessive terminal androgen-dependent hair with a typical male distribution. This commonly involves chin, upper lip, side of the face, breasts, lower abdomen and thighs. Such a distribution of hair may be accepted as normal by some cultures but equally may be a sign of a serious endocrine abnormality that requires further investigation and treatment. This is particularly so if hirsutism is associated with signs of virilisation, namely clitoral hypertrophy, temporal hair recession and breast atrophy.

Except for the palms and soles, hair follicles are present virtually throughout the body. Hair growth in women occurs in the following major areas:

1. *Pubic (lower escutcheon)* and *axillary hair* are androgen-dependent and their follicles clearly have androgen receptors but do not appear to require testosterone [or more important, its metabolite dihydrotestosterone (DHT)] to stimulate them. Pubic hair appears some 2 years before the onset of axillary hair growth and appears in girls at a mean age of 13.7 years, compared with 15.2 years in their male counterparts. Considerable evidence suggests that it is adrenal androgen production that is responsible for the initial production of lower escutcheon pubic and axillary hair.

2. *Facial hair, body hair (including upper pubic escutcheon)* and *sebaceous glands* are also androgen-dependent but appear to require the conversion of testosterone to DHT by the enzyme 5α-reductase to convert fine vellus hair to terminal hair and to increase the rate of sebum secretion by sebaceous glands (Fig. 3.2). This results in the development of characteristic male pattern hair on the face, chest, upper male pubic escutcheon and limbs as well as the development of a greasy skin (sebum is rich in lipid) and acne. The enzyme 5α-reductase in hair follicles is dependent on testosterone so that it is induced by its own substrate. In contrast 5α-reductase in the genital skin is independent of circulating testosterone levels. DHT is metabolised by skin to inactive androstanediol. Whilst thigh hair is a male characteristic there is less of a sexual difference in hair on the upper limbs.

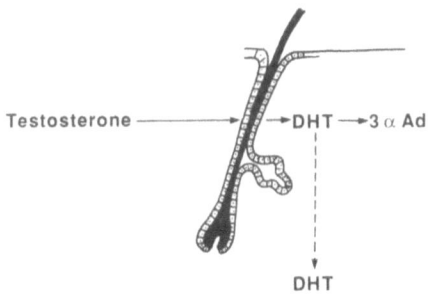

Fig. 3.2. Metabolism of testosterone by the hair follicle. Whilst DHT is the active androgen, most of it is metabolised locally (*continuous lines*) and only small amounts reach the blood (*dotted line*), so that plasma DHT is a poor reflection of peripheral conversion of testosterone. The estimation of androstanediol (3αAd) correlates much better with the degree of hirsutism.

3. *Scalp hair* differs from all other hair in that its growth is not androgen-dependent but paradoxically it appears that hair loss in genetically predisposed subjects may be androgen-mediated, terminal hair being converted to a vellus pattern.

That each hair reaches a definitive length and then stops growing is a consequence of the hair cycle (Fig. 3.3). During active growth (anagen) the hair is formed from epidermal cells which are invaginated by a dermal papilla

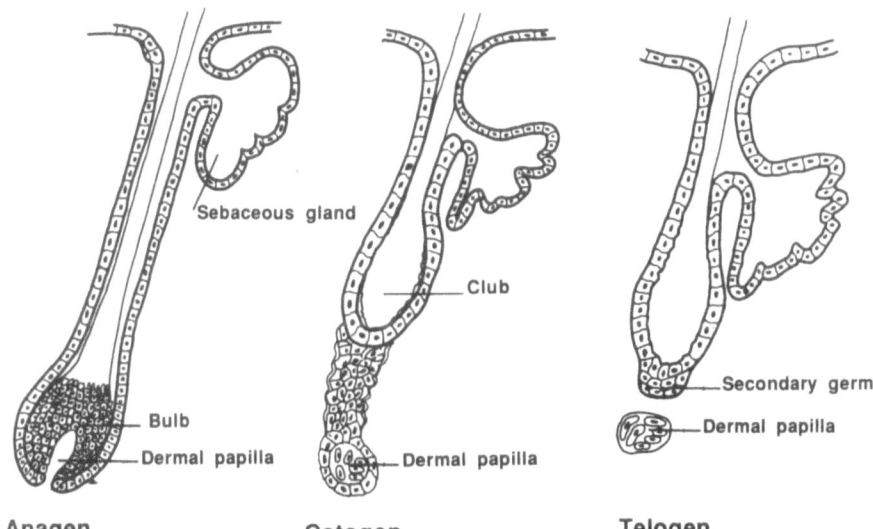

Fig. 3.3. The human hair cycle.

to form the hair bulb. Melanocytes then add pigment to the proliferating cells. The termination of this phase is marked by a reduction in pigmentation, the middle region of the bulb becomes constricted and the base of the hair expands and is keratinised to form a club (catagen). The club hair moves distally with a column of epidermal cells (secondary germ) releasing the dermal papilla. The secondary germ is in a resting phase (telogen) and the club hair is retained until a newly active follicle is formed from the secondary germ, when it is moulted. The average rate of hair growth ranges from 0.2 mm per day for hair on the thighs to 0.5 mm per day for hair on the scalp. Anagen may last for up to 3 months for body hair and 3 years for scalp hair. At any one time approximately 86% of hair follicles are in anagen, 13% in telogen and 1% in catagen.

All hair follicles have the capacity to differentiate into either terminal hair or a sebaceous follicle, in which the sebaceous gland becomes prominent and the hair remains vellus. Terminal hairs are wider, longer and darker than vellus hairs. Androgens are the principal factor determining the production of terminal rather than vellus hair and they also increase the proportion of the time spent in anagen. Thus the only difference in sexual hair in men and women is the mass of hair converted to terminal hair. Therefore, with rising androgen levels in puberty and in pathophysiological states of hyperandrogen production, there is increased recruitment of hair follicles to terminal hair in accordance with a preset genetic sensitivity to androgen. Thus genital and pubic hair is more sensitive than body hair which in turn is more sensitive than scalp hair. In the United Kingdom the incidence of terminal hair growth for women is 18% on the chest, 28% on the cheeks, 35% on the abdomen and 70% on the limbs.

Androgens reaching hair follicles in the female are DHA, its sulphate (DHAS), androstenedione and testosterone following secretion by the adrenal gland and the ovary. Furthermore, weak androgens such as androstenedione may be converted by peripheral tissues such as fat to the more potent androgen testosterone by the enzyme aromatase. The fetal ovary is relatively inactive but the fetal adrenal secretes significant quantities of DHA, DHAS, androstenedione and testosterone. However, the secretion of these sex steroids declines markedly after birth and until puberty there is little androgen secretion. As puberty approaches, the adrenal secretion of androgens increases (adrenarche). The mechanism is unknown but is independent of gonadotrophins and probably involves maturation of the zones producing sex steroids—the adrenocortical fasciculata and reticularis. The adrenarche occurs in boys at 6–7 years of age and in girls at 8–9 years, preceding the gonadarche at 10–12 years in girls and 12–14 years in boys; both events are independent phenomena. The adrenarche is probably responsible for the stimulation of pubic and axillary hair growth.

Following the menarche there is an ovarian contribution to sex-steroid production. At this stage of development, 90% of DHAS is due to adrenal secretion with 10% derived from peripheral conversion and none from the ovary. Fifty per cent of DHA is derived from the adrenal with 30% from peripheral conversion and 20% from the ovary. Fifty per cent of androstenedione is derived from the adrenal with 50% from the ovary although the ovarian contribution increases during ovulation. The relative contributions of the most physiologically active androgen, testosterone, are approximately 33% each from adrenal, peripheral conversion and ovary. Following the menopause 50% of women continue to secrete significant amounts of testosterone.

Testosterone is transported in blood by sex-hormone-binding globulin (SHBG) (68%) and to a lesser extent by albumin (30%) leaving 2% as a free fraction. Whilst it is traditionally thought that it is the free hormone that is the biologically active fraction, recent evidence suggests that the albumin-bound fraction is also available to some tissues.

Diagnosis

The pathophysiology of abnormal androgen secretion in hirsute women can be regarded as a spectrum without sharp borderlines from normal to non-tumorous conditions, such as idiopathic hirsutism and polycystic ovarian syndrome, through to tumours of the ovary and adrenal. Excessive secretion of DHT, testosterone, androstenedione and DHA is often derived from mixed sources and dynamic function tests do not discriminate reliably between the various causes. However, it is only testosterone, particularly the free testosterone, and not the levels of the other androgens, that correlates with the degree of hirsutism. The failure of DHT to correlate with the degree of hirsutism can be explained by its metabolism to androstanediol by the hair follicle. 5α-Reductase activity is significantly increased in hirsute women and this enzyme may be the key factor in the development of hirsutism.

1. In *idiopathic hirsutism* plasma androgen levels are raised when patients are considered as a group and compared with normals, but raised androgens in peripheral blood are evident only in 60% of patients when hormone analysis is restricted to plasma DHAS and testosterone. However, plasma SHBG levels in these patients are often reduced, increasing the free testosterone available to the hair follicles. Furthermore there is increased utilisation of testosterone in these patients by increased 5α-reductase activity. The cause of this increased activity is unclear but induction of the enzyme may have occurred during puberty. In these patients plasma levels of 3α-androstanediol gluconuride are elevated confirming increased 5α-reductase activity.

2. It is debatable whether the *polycystic ovarian syndrome* is a separate entity from idiopathic hirsutism but it most probably represents a continuing spectrum of increased androgen production with raised levels of free testosterone, androstenedione, DHA and DHAS. In these patients there is evidence of abnormalities of the hypothalamus and pituitary with suppressed FSH and elevated LH levels and menstrual disturbance. The ovarian anatomical abnormalities characteristic of the disorder are usually microscopic but can be detected by ultrasonography in good hands. However, they are

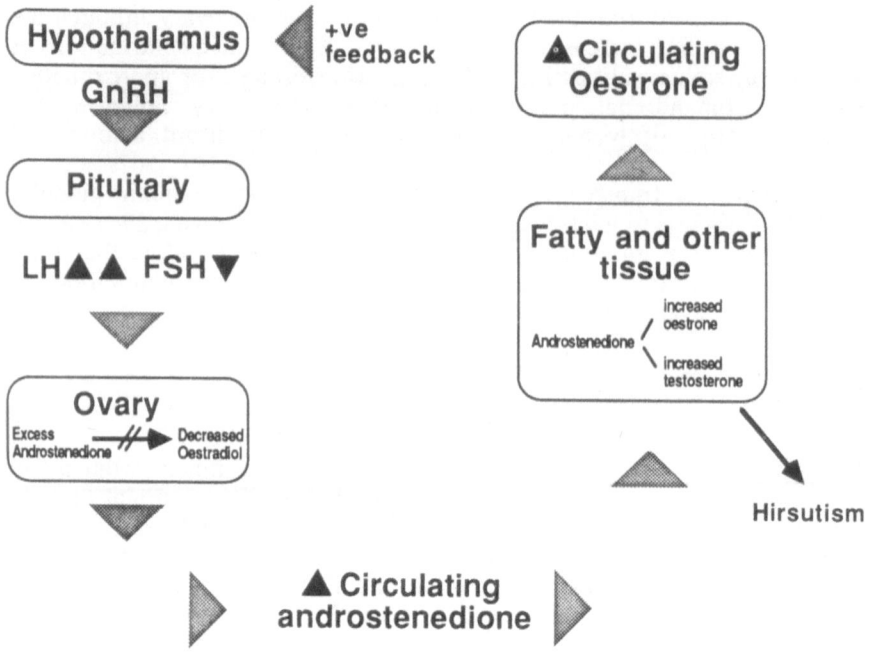

Fig. 3.4. The pathogenesis of the polycystic ovarian syndrome (see text for details).

rarely clinically palpable as in the classic Stein–Leventhal syndrome. Whether these abnormalities are primary or secondary has not been established. Hypersecretion of androgens from mixed ovarian/adrenal origin with subsequent peripheral conversion to oestrogen (principally oestrone) as well as testosterone probably results in the abnormal pattern of gonadotrophins with raised LH levels (positive feedback) and suppressed FSH (negative feedback). This abnormal pattern leads to failure of ovulation and to polycystic ovaries. Polycystic ovaries secrete abnormal amounts of androgen to maintain a vicious cycle (Fig. 3.4). What initiates events is unknown but may reflect increased androgen production from an abnormal adrenarche.

Idiopathic hirsutism and polycystic ovarian syndrome account for the majority of cases of hirsutism and the other causes are extremely uncommon.

Treatment

The identification and localisation of androgen-secreting tumours is of the utmost importance. Plasma testosterone and DHAS appear to be the most useful markers since androgen-secreting ovarian and adrenal tumours hardly ever occur without elevation of either of these hormones in peripheral blood.

A tumour must be suspected in a patient with a rapid onset of virilisation and raised plasma levels of testosterone (>1.5 ng/ml or 5.2 nmol/l) and DHAS (> 9000 ng/ml or 23 mmol/l). These patients should undergo selective venous catheterisation of ovarian and adrenal veins to determine the gradients of androgen secretion and subsequent localisation of the tumour. Computerised tomography is a useful adjunct when an adrenal tumour is indicated. Appropriate treatment is removal of the tumour.

Women with mild, early onset, non-progressive hirsutism and plasma testosterone and DHAS levels <1.5 ng/ml or 5.2 nmol/l and <9000 ng/ml or 23 mmol/l respectively do not require catheter studies. A diagnosis of polycystic ovarian syndrome can be confirmed if necessary by estimation of plasma gonadotrophins and pelvic ultrasound. If the hirsutism is only mild to moderate no therapy other than reassurance may be required. Local measures such as shaving and electrolysis can be recommended and there is no evidence that shaving increases the rate of hair growth. However, plucking the hair should be avoided as this stimulates a new anagen phase. For patients with appreciable and understandable social embarrassment, medical therapy may be offered after discussing the risks of treatment weighed against any likely benefit. In particular, it should be stressed that a response is unlikely to occur before 3 months (the average anagen phase of body hair) and that hirsutism will recur on withdrawal of therapy, which will therefore have to be continued indefinitely. Medical treatment can be divided into three groups:

1. The administration of *glucocorticoid* in such a manner to cause adrenal suppression can be successful at reducing plasma testosterone levels but also probably acts by direct suppression of the ovary as well. Dexamethasone 0.5–1.0 mg given last thing at night should achieve suppression of the pituitary–adrenal axis although an impaired response to stress may be an undesirable consequence.

2. *Cyproterone acetate* is an anti-androgen exerting its effect, in part, by acting as a competitive antagonist of testosterone and DHT. Since the drug has progestogen-like activity and a prolonged half-life it is given with oestrogen in a reversed sequential regimen. Ethinyloestradiol 50 µg daily from days 5 to 21 of the menstrual cycle should be given with cyproterone acetate 100 mg daily from days 5 to 15 of the cycle. This treatment is given cyclically. The regimen is effective in about 70% of patients and probably contraceptive, but has the side-effects of cyproterone acetate and the risks associated with the prolonged use of oral oestrogen. It is important that the patient is told that pregnancy must be avoided, as a male fetus could be exposed to an anti-androgen in utero. In children there is evidence that cyproterone acetate may cause adrenal suppression but this does not appear to be the case in adults. However, this drug may cause a marked loss of libido.

3. The oral administration of *spironolactone* 50–75 mg daily suppresses testosterone synthesis and inhibits the enzyme 5α-reductase, achieving improvement in 80% of patients with few side-effects. Any abnormal uterine bleeding in mid-cycle should be treated with the addition of an oral contraceptive agent.

If fertility is a problem in patients with polycystic ovarian syndrome, induction of ovulation may be attempted.

1. *Clomiphene citrate* will usually induce ovulation in 80% of patients with a conception rate of 35% within three cycles. Those who fail to conceive should be treated with gonadotrophin therapy as success with pulsatile GnRH therapy in this group is poor.

2. *Gonadotrophin therapy* in patients with polycystic ovarian syndrome differs from that in patients with secondary ovarian failure. In polycystic ovarian syndrome one of the major abnormalities is increased secretion of LH relative to FSH by the anterior pituitary. Menotrophin consists of equal amounts of FSH to LH and will not correct the abnormal gonadotrophin profile found in polycystic patients.

Instead of menotrophin, a pure preparation of FSH should be employed for the induction of follicular development. Urofollitropin (human menopausal FSH) is given by intramuscular injection in a dose of 75–150 units daily and the response monitored by the estimation of plasma oestradiol and ovarian ultrasound in the usual way. As soon as adequate follicular development has been achieved, a single dose of 10 000 units hCG is given intramuscularly. The cumulative conception rate in these patients who have previously failed on clomiphene is 50% after five cycles and 75% after 12 cycles.

4 The Testis

As in the female, the anterior pituitary secretion of LH and FSH in the male is under the control of the pulsatile hypothalamic release of GnRH. With the start of male puberty, plasma LH levels rise progressively, first during the night and later during the day as well. LH is released in a pulsatile manner at approximately 90-minute intervals. Stimulated by LH, the Leydig cells of the testis secrete testosterone which exerts negative feedback inhibition over LH secretion at the level of the hypothalamus and the anterior pituitary. FSH in combination with the local production of testosterone stimulates spermatogenesis, and enlargement of the testis during puberty is mainly attributable to growth of the seminiferous tubules. Spermatogenesis is associated with the production of inhibin which selectively inhibits the anterior pituitary secretion of FSH.

Testosterone circulates in the plasma largely bound to the plasma proteins sex-hormone-binding globulin (SHBG, 44%) and albumin (54%) and only 2% is free (the biologically active fraction). The concentration of SHBG in the plasma is regulated by several hormones and is increased by oestrogens, hyperthyroidism and hypogonadism; levels are decreased by hypothyroidism. Testosterone is metabolised by the enzyme 5α-reductase to its active metabolite dihydrotestosterone (DHT, 8%) and by the enzyme aromatase to oestradiol (0.3%); the majority (90%) is excreted in the urine as inactive metabolites. Testosterone is responsible for regulation of gonadotrophin secretion and the development of the Wolffian ducts during male sexual differentiation, whereas DHT is responsible for the development of male external genitalia during embryogenesis and male secondary sex characteristics during puberty. The secretion of oestrogen by the testis and its peripheral conversion from testosterone account for the gynaecomastia that sometimes occurs during puberty (prolactin is not involved).

Hypogonadism

Diagnosis

Hypogonadism with Raised Plasma Gonadotrophins

Primary gonadal failure usually presents with symptoms of androgen deficiency (reduced libido, impotence and redistribution of body fat to a female pattern) and can be confirmed by the finding of low plasma testosterone concentrations and elevated plasma gonadotrophin concentrations. There are several causes:

1. Physiological testicular failure occurs with age but does not normally develop until after the age of 50 years.

2. Gonadal dysgenesis and chromosome abnormalities present with failure of pubertal development. If the problem is one of gonadal dysgenesis the internal and external genital structures will be female and the patient will complain of primary amenorrhoea. If the problem is one of a chromosome abnormality in a phenotypic male (Klinefelter's syndrome, XXY), failure of normal androgen production in childhood results in continued growth of long bones so that span exceeds height and the lower body segment exceeds the upper segment (eunuchoid proportion). The external genitalia fail to mature, pubic hair is confined to the lower triangle, body fat is distributed in the female pattern and there is gynaecomastia.

3. Autoimmune testicular destruction may be associated with Addison's disease in the same way as primary ovarian failure.

4. Miscellaneous causes include cytotoxic drugs and irradiation. Viruses such as mumps rarely cause testicular failure and bilateral cryptorchidism is usually associated with normal testosterone production but impaired spermatogenesis.

Hypogonadism with Normal or Low Plasma Gonadotrophin Concentrations

Secondary gonadal failure occurs in three major contexts:

1. Weight-related hypogonadism is much less common in males than in their female counterparts but anorexia nervosa, when it does occur, produces a regression of gonadotrophin secretion to a prepubertal pattern.

2. Isolated GnRH deficiency occurs in males in the same way as in females (Kallmann's syndrome).

3. Pituitary and parapituitary lesions including hyperprolactinaemia are discussed in Chapter 5.

4. Delayed puberty cannot easily be distinguished from GnRH insufficiency except in retrospect.

Treatment

Primary testicular failure should be treated with sex hormone replacement therapy. Testosterone may be given by three routes (Fig. 4.1):

1. *Testosterone undecanoate* is the only effective orally active testosterone (other preparations are inactivated by the liver) and may be given in a dose of 40–80 mg 12-hourly. Although this route of administration avoids the need for parenteral therapy, most patients are dissatisfied with this form of treatment compared with the other two alternatives. It is also very expensive.

2. *Testosterone esters* can be given by intramuscular injection as Sustanon 250 (Organon), containing a mixture of testosterone propionate 30 mg, testosterone phenylpropionate 60 mg, testosterone isocaproate 60 mg and testosterone decanoate 100 mg in 1 ml of oily vehicle to be administered every 3–4 weeks. This route is preferred by many patients to the oral route, as it avoids the need for a twice-daily tablet regimen. However, it produces wide fluctuations in plasma testosterone concentrations and may be less physiological than testosterone implants.

3. *Testosterone implantation* is usually achieved by the subcutaneous administration of 600 mg testosterone in the form of six 100 mg pellets introduced into the anterior abdominal wall by means of a trocar under local anaesthetic and aseptic conditions. Despite the apparent trauma of this method it is the route preferred by many patients as it provides sustained levels of plasma testosterone concentrations for a period of up to 6 months.

Treatment of secondary testicular failure should be directed at the underlying cause (treatment of hyperprolactinaemia is discussed in Chapter 5) but irreversible androgen deficiency may be treated by testosterone replacement therapy. However, if fertility is required, induction of spermatogenesis may be attempted by the following means:

1. *Gonadotrophin therapy* involves the stimulation of testosterone secretion from the Leydig cells by the intramuscular administration of hCG 1500 units twice weekly. Spermatogenesis is induced by the concomitant intramuscular administration of menotrophin (human menopausal gonadotrophin containing equal amounts of LH and FSH) 150 units three times weekly. The response should be monitored by monthly estimation of plasma testosterone, plasma oestradiol and semen analysis. If plasma oestradiol levels exceed the normal male range (150 pmol/l) the dose of hCG should be reduced as increased testicular production of oestrogen may inhibit spermatogenesis. No increase in the sperm count should be expected for several months and treatment has to be continued for a minimum period of 6 months.

2. *Pulsatile GnRH therapy* is gradually replacing gonadotrophin therapy for the treatment of infertility due to hypogonadotrophic hypogonadism. GnRH is administered in a dose of approximately 5 μg subcutaneously every 90 minutes via a portable pump. The response should be monitored by

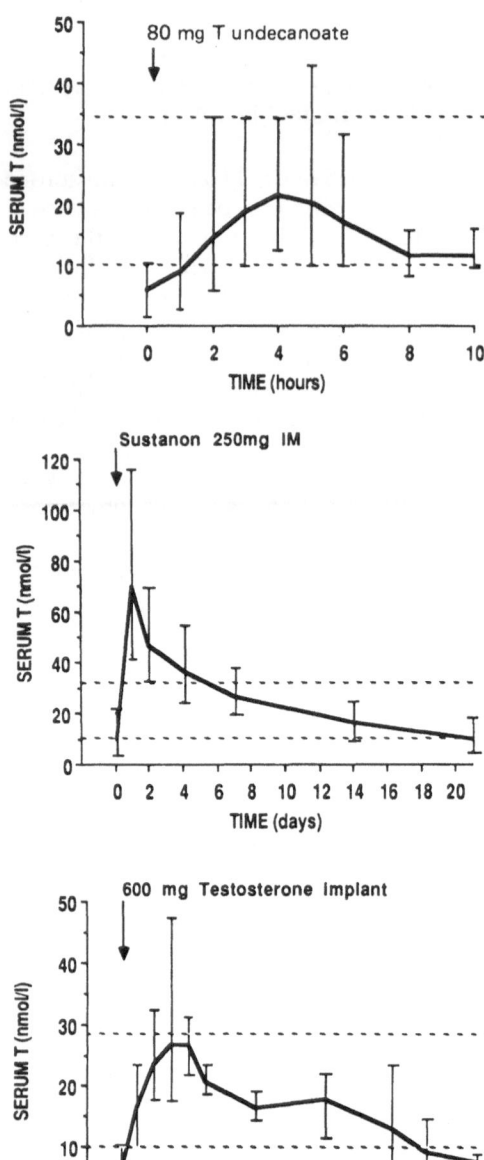

Fig. 4.1. Serum testosterone (T) concentrations following the administration of either oral testosterone undecanoate 80 mg, intramuscular testosterone 250 mg or testosterone 600 mg by implant. The dashed lines indicate the normal reference range for serum testosterone concentrations. (From Cantrill JA et al. (1984) *Clin Endocrinol* 21: 97–107.)

estimation of plasma testosterone concentrations and semen analysis; treatment should be continued for at least 6 months.

Hypergonadism: Precocious Puberty

Diagnosis

Sexual development before the age of 9 years in boys is considered abnormal and may be brought about by two different causes:

1. *Virilising syndromes* result from excessive production of androgens from Leydig cell tumours or hyperplasia, GnRH- or hCG-secreting tumours, congenital adrenal hyperplasia (see Chapter 2) or androgen administration. In true idiopathic precocious puberty there is activation of the pituitary–gonadal axis with both LH and FSH secretion, and hence spermatogenesis, whereas in pseudo-precocious puberty, spermatogenesis is absent.

2. *Premature activation of the hypothalamic–pituitary axis* (idiopathic precocious puberty) may have its onset in infancy and is heralded by testicular enlargement associated with nocturnal pubertal patterns of LH secretion and eventually adult plasma testosterone concentrations. The mechanism of the initiation of normal puberty is ill understood and it is therefore not surprising that the pathogenesis of precocious puberty is unknown.

Treatment

Treatment of virilising syndromes should be directed at the underlying disorder. The management of idiopathic precocious puberty is generally unsatisfactory, but recently the administration of long-acting analogues of GnRH has proved promising with "down-regulation" of anterior pituitary gonadotrophin receptors and suppression of both plasma LH and testosterone concentrations.

5 The Pituitary Gland

THE ANTERIOR PITUITARY

The anterior pituitary gland synthesises and secretes growth hormone (hGH), prolactin (PRL), gonadotrophins (LH and FSH), thyrotrophin (TSH) and corticotrophin (ACTH).

Growth hormone, which has a plasma half-life of approximately 25 minutes, is secreted by the anterior pituitary and stimulates skeletal and soft tissue growth. This is associated with positive nitrogen balance and positive calcium balance, although increased intestinal absorption of calcium may lead to hypercalciuria and increased urinary loss of calcium. Some effects of hGH are mediated indirectly by acting on the liver, as its target organ, to stimulate the synthesis and secretion of the somatomedins. The somatomedins share a degree of homology with proinsulin and two somatomedins have been identified with two different receptors: IGF I and IGF II (insulin-like growth factors).

IGF I is measured in the blood by a radioimmunoassay that is available to some routine laboratories and concentrations are relatively constant throughout the day. However, levels of IGF I change as a function of age, being low before the age of 6 years, rising through childhood and rising steeply in association with puberty. Pubertal levels are approximately twice those in the adult and fall to a plasma concentration that remains relatively constant from the age of 20 until old age. Blood levels of IGF I are undetectable in cases of hGH deficiency and elevated in cases of hGH excess. In contrast, IGF II is less hGH-dependent; it is reduced in cases of hGH deficiency, but changes little with hGH excess.

Secretion of hGH is under the control of two hypothalamic peptides: GH-releasing hormone (GHRH) and GH-inhibiting hormone (somatostatin). Control of anterior pituitary hGH secretion is complex involving negative feedback and neural control mechanisms. At the level of the hypothalamus both hGH and IGF I stimulate somatostatin and thereby inhibit hGH release and at the level of the anterior pituitary somatotroph IGF

I is inhibitory. The neuronal systems regulating GHRH and somatostatin receive a variety of neuronal inputs. Secretion of hGH is increased during sleep and by hypoglycaemia and exercise. The secretion of GHRH is stimulated by acetylcholine, α-adrenergic and dopaminergic stimuli and inhibited by β-adrenergic stimuli. In the pathological state of acromegaly, TRH, GnRH and glucose may stimulate hGH secretion, and plasma hGH levels are elevated in anorexia nervosa and starvation. Human GH levels are low in the plasma in the early postnatal months and during early childhood are similar to adult levels. During puberty there is an increase in the frequency and amplitude of hGH pulses. The most marked changes occur at night, with paroxysmal hGH secretion starting approximately 1 hour after the onset of sleep. Plasma hGH levels are routinely measured by radioimmunoassay.

Prolactin acts directly on the breast but has little role in breast development and is responsible for the initiation and development of lactation. The action of prolactin on lactation requires priming of the breast tissue with oestrogens and progesterone. Paradoxically, during pregnancy lactation is inhibited by the high levels of oestrogen and progesterone and it is following delivery that oestrogen levels fall allowing the unopposed action of prolactin to stimulate lactation. Prolactin in excess acts through the dopaminergic and opioid mechanisms of the hypothalamus to inhibit GnRH secretion to produce a hypogonadotrophic hypogonadism. The hormone may also have a direct action by suppressing gonadal function. The secretion of prolactin is controlled by the hypothalamic secretion of dopamine which inhibits its release. In contrast TRH stimulates prolactin secretion in pharmacological amounts but its physiological importance is unknown. Suckling is another potent stimulus for prolactin release. Prolactin is measured routinely by radioimmunoassay.

The control and secretion of TSH, ACTH and gonadotrophins have been discussed in previous chapters.

Hypopituitarism

Diagnosis

Hypopituitarism may result from a wide variety of hypothalamic or pituitary diseases. In some cases there may be an isolated deficiency of one pituitary hormone. More commonly several, if not all (panhypopituitarism), anterior pituitary hormones may be lost. This latter most often occurs with progressive expansion of a macroadenoma. Deficiency of hGH is often the first indication of developing pituitary failure followed by LH, FSH, TSH and ACTH deficiencies. Prolactin secretion is often well preserved unless there has been pituitary infarction following post-partum haemorrhage. Other causes of hypopituitarism include autoimmune hypophysitis, granulomatous conditions (such as sarcoidosis, Wegner's granulomatosis and histiocytosis-X), vascular disturbance and metastatic carcinoma.

If the plasma cortisol level is within the normal 09.00 hours range, there is no history of epilepsy or ischaemic heart disease and the ECG is normal then anterior pituitary function is tested by the combined intravenous administration of insulin (0.15 U soluble insulin/kg body weight), TRH (200 µg) and GnRH (50 µg). Cortisol, glucose and hGH levels are measured at 0, 30, 60, 90 and 120 minutes; PRL, TSH, LH and FSH at 0, 30 and 60 minutes. The insulin test depends on adequate hypoglycaemia being achieved (blood glucose <2 mmol/l). Hypopituitarism is considered if:

1. The peak hGH response is less than 20 mU/l.
2. The LH increment is less than four times basal levels (absolute peak LH <10 U/l) and the FSH increment less than one and a half times basal levels (absolute peak <5 U/l for females and <2 U/l for males). In addition plasma oestradiol should be estimated in women and testosterone in men. Ovulation in women is best assessed by estimation of plasma progesterone (ovulation >20 nmol/l) levels on day 21 of the menstrual cycle.
3. The peak TSH level is less than 3.0 mU/l at 30 minutes and 3.0 mU/l at 60 minutes. In addition plasma thyroid hormones should be measured.
4. The peak cortisol level is less than 550 nmol/l.
5. In patients with prolactin-secreting tumours there may be an impaired prolactin response to TRH but this is not necessarily diagnostic.

Treatment

Panhypopituitarism is treated by replacement with hydrocortisone (20 mg before breakfast and 10 mg at 18.00 hours), L-thyroxine (usually 0.15 mg daily) and sex hormones as appropriate. Mineralocorticoid replacement therapy is not required as patients with hypopituitarism have an intact renin–angiotensin system that can maintain normal aldosterone secretion. In men testosterone is replaced by the monthly intramuscular injection of testosterone esters (Sustanon 250 mg) or by subcutaneous implantation of testosterone (200–600 mg) every 6 months. In women cyclical oestrogen and progesterone therapy should be initiated if appropriate. In children growth failure can be treated by the administration of GH by injection (Fig. 5.1). Until recently GH was extracted from post-mortem pituitaries but this source has been discontinued because of possible slow-virus contamination. Recombinant DNA technology, however, has now resulted in an abundant supply of GH available for use. It is usually given in a dose of 10 units intramuscularly twice weekly although some centres are now giving more frequent subcutaneous injections. Response to this therapy is carefully monitored in terms of growth velocity. In the first year of treatment the growth velocity should increase two- to fourfold from 3.6 to 9.4 cm/yr. Over succeeding years the growth velocity tends to fall off. Long-term results of treatment suggest that height lost in childhood is not necessarily recovered.

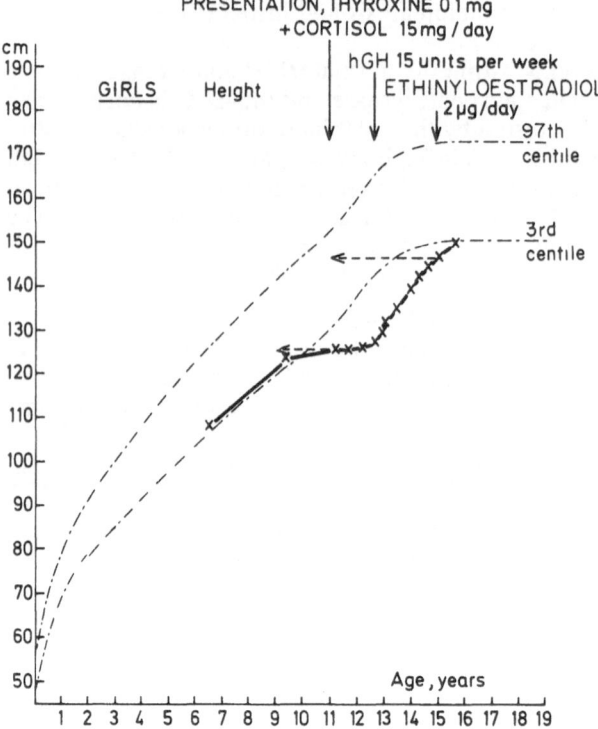

Fig. 5.1. Human GH (hGH) therapy in the treatment of hypopituitarism. Care must be taken in instituting corticosteroid replacement and sex-steroid therapy otherwise premature fusion of the epiphyses may develop (*arrows* indicate bone age). The figure shows data for girls.

In patients with isolated hGH deficiency the final height attained is usually two standard deviations below the mean and, whilst this is significantly better than the six standard deviations below the mean found in untreated cases, only 50% of males and 15% of females manage to reach the third centile. In patients with hypopituitarism the response is better with a final height of one standard deviation below the mean. However, in these cases improved final height results in body disproportion with long legs, the severity of which is related to the age of starting sex-hormone replacement. Care must be taken in order to ensure that the patient with hypopituitarism is receiving adequate replacement with L-thyroxine and that the dose of glucocorticoid is not excessive, otherwise growth will be inhibited. Sex-steroid replacement requires careful timing so that premature fusion of epiphyses is avoided and adequate advantage is taken of the synergy between sex steroids and hGH.

GH-releasing hormone will probably be used in the future for the treatment of children with isolated hGH deficiency, a defect caused by a deficiency of GHRH. This may be given subcutaneously by a small portable pump to mimic the natural pulsatile secretion of hGH. Initial results with this treatment have been promising. Similarly, puberty and fertility may be induced in some patients by the pulsatile administration of GnRH.

Pituitary Tumours

Pituitary tumours produce a constellation of symptoms and signs that indicate either a direct effect of tumour expansion upon surrounding structures, or inappropriate or defective secretion of pituitary hormones.

Diagnosis

Pituitary tumours can be classified according to anatomical size and function. Previous histological classifications are outmoded and have little clinical use. On the basis of computerised tomography, pituitary tumours may be divided into two groups:

1. *Microadenomas* are less than 10 mm in diameter and fail to distort the pituitary fossa or cause hypopituitarism.

2. *Macroadenomas* obviously distort the sella contours and may extend outside the anatomical bounds of the pituitary fossa. Local effects include headaches resulting from progressive expansion of a tumour within the sella turcica, stretching the diaphragma sellae and eroding the pituitary fossa. The local anatomy of the pituitary is initially assessed by plain skull radiography (postero-anterior and lateral) (Fig. 5.2) and careful charting of the visual fields using a Bjerrum screen or the Goldman apparatus (Fig. 5.3). Cranial nerve palsies are important clinical signs of extension. Suprasellar extension can compromise the optic pathways and cause visual field impairment. Lateral extension into the cavernous sinus is indicated by III, IV or VI nerve palsies. The suprasellar region may be more accurately assessed by computerised tomography or positive contrast cisternography. An enlarged sella turcica can also be occupied by cerebrospinal fluid (empty sella syndrome). In the primary form, a defect in the diaphragma sellae allows transmission of cerebrospinal fluid pressure waves to expand and erode the pituitary fossa. Headaches are a common symptom, but hypopituitarism is infrequent. In the secondary form, a pre-existing pituitary tumour either undergoes infarction or shrinks as a result of therapy. In both primary and

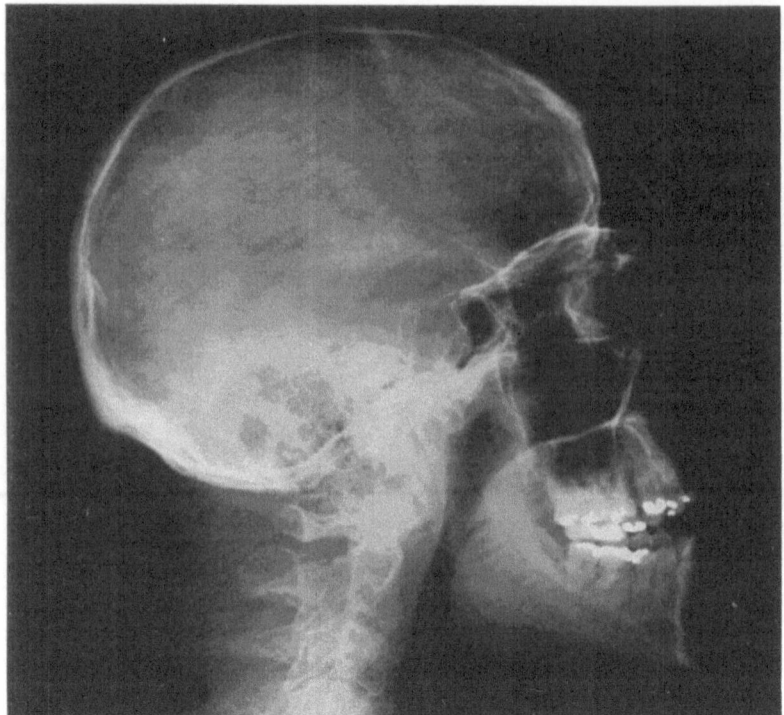

Fig. 5.2. Plain skull radiography to illustrate a macroadenoma of the pituitary gland.

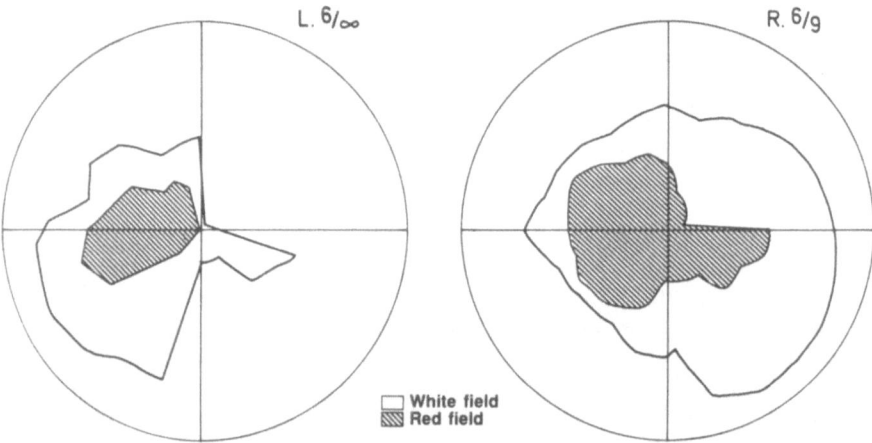

Fig. 5.3. Careful charting of the visual fields is vital in patients with a pituitary tumour. Colour vision (red light) is affected more than white and any pattern of visual field defect may occur depending on the direction of growth of the tumour in relation to the visual pathways.

secondary forms there is a risk of prolapse of the optic nerves into the sella turcica, causing visual failure and field defects. Carotid angiography is a wise precaution prior to neurosurgery as expansion of the sella turcica may rarely result from an intracranial aneurysm.

Pituitary tumours may also be defined according to the type of hormone that is secreted.

1. *Prolactin-secreting tumours* are the commonest tumours of the anterior pituitary accounting for 32% of cases. The majority of women present in early reproductive life with amenorrhoea and infertility. However, any type of menstrual abnormality may be associated with hyperprolactinaemia. The incidence of galactorrhoea is variable (30%–80%) and visual field impairment due to an expanding tumour is fortunately uncommon (10%). Men present with impotence (90%) and obesity (50%). Galactorrhoea is unusual but many patients have evidence of suprasellar expansion often reflecting the delay in diagnosis of a prolactinoma as the cause of impotence. Hyperprolactinaemia is not always attributable to a prolactinoma. Only after exclusion of pregnancy, prolactin-stimulating drugs, renal failure and hypothyroidism can the diagnosis be entertained. With high prolactin levels (above 2000 mU/l) a confident diagnosis of a macroprolactinoma can be made if the pituitary fossa is obviously enlarged on plain skull radiography. The diagnosis of a microprolactinoma is more difficult. The pituitary fossa is not obviously enlarged and the differential diagnosis rests between prolactinoma, hypothalamic disease and idiopathic hyperplasia of prolactin-secreting cells. Plasma prolactin levels in excess of 2000 mU/l are strongly suggestive of a microprolactinoma, but the diagnosis can also be entertained for lower levels.

2. *Growth-hormone-secreting tumours* account for 27% of anterior pituitary tumours including 10% which also secrete prolactin. Hypersecretion of hGH by a pituitary adenoma leads to excessive growth of the soft tissues and skeleton. Rarely, this occurs prior to fusion of the epiphyses and results in gigantism. In the adult, symptoms and signs of acromegaly develop insidiously over many years and the gradual change in appearance is often evident when old photographs are reviewed. The diagnosis of hGH hypersecretion rests on the failure of plasma hGH levels to suppress in response to a glucose load. Blood is taken at 30-minute intervals for 2 hours for the estimation of whole blood glucose and plasma GH levels following the oral administration of 75 g glucose. Normal individuals should suppress plasma hGH to a level of <2 mU/l.

3. *Corticotrophin-secreting tumours* account for 13% of anterior pituitary tumours and the diagnosis of Cushing's disease has already been discussed.

4. *Non-functioning pituitary adenomas* account for 23% of anterior pituitary tumours. These tumours fail to secrete either prolactin, hGH, ACTH, TSH or gonadotrophin. Symptoms and signs result from the local consequences of tumour expansion.

5. *Other types of tumour* are rare, namely TSH- and gonadotrophin-secreting tumours, accounting for 5% of anterior pituitary tumours.

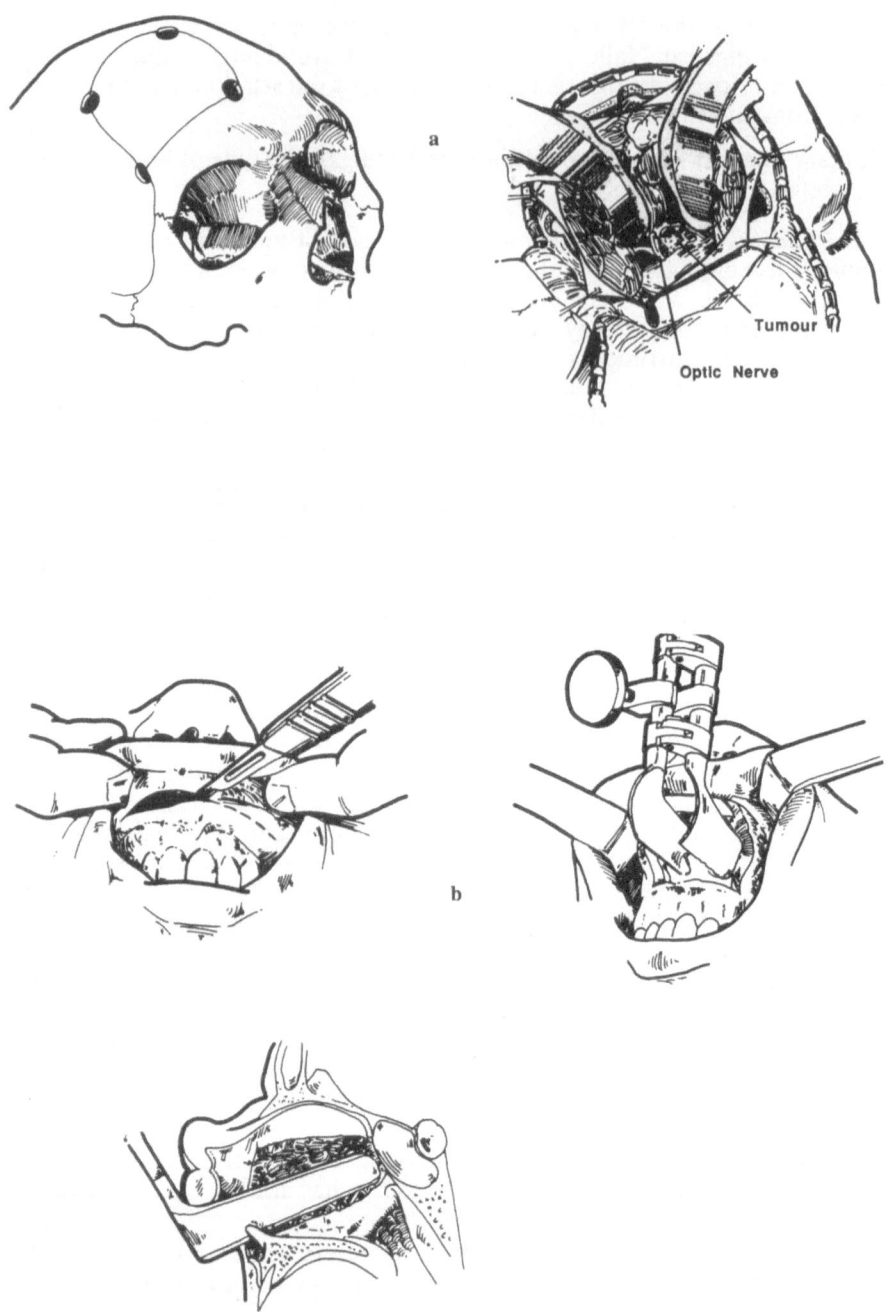

Fig. 5.4. The neurosurgical approaches to the pituitary gland: transfrontal craniotomy (**a**) and transsphenoidal (**b**).

Treatment

Pituitary tumours can be treated by surgery, radiotherapy or by medical means.

1. *Surgical access* to the pituitary is gained either by a frontal craniotomy or by the transsphenoidal route (Fig. 5.4). The transsphenoidal operation has several attractions and is suitable for almost all patients. It can achieve an effective and radical decompression in the majority of patients who have a large tumour even if there is large suprasellar extension. After evacuation of the tumour the diaphragma sellae descends from the suprasellar cistern into the vacant space in the fossa under positive intracranial pressure. This approach avoids complications specific to the intracranial route including intracranial haematoma, and a 5% risk of epilepsy.

2. *Radiotherapy* is usually administered by external pituitary irradiation using a conventional linear accelerator or less commonly by yttrium-90 implantation. In some centres external irradiation is given through two opposed temporal fields to a total dose of 3750 cGy over 15 fractions in 21 days. Other centres use a third field with an increased number of fractions whilst maintaining a similar total dose (not exceeding 4500 cGy) in an attempt to reduce the radiation dose per fraction and the total dose to the temporal lobes. However, the former method is simple, effective and apparently without serious side-effects. A relatively high incidence of hypopituitarism is a complication of both methods.

3. *Medical treatment* in the form of dopamine agonist drugs has revolutionised the treatment of prolactinomas. Bromocriptine is introduced cautiously in a dose of 1.25 mg orally with a snack on going to bed as it may cause severe postural hypotension, nausea and vomiting. On waking the next day the patient can take a further 1.25 mg if there were no adverse side-effects and the dose gradually increased to 2.5 mg 8-hourly for the treatment of prolactinomas and 5–10 mg 8-hourly for hGH-secreting tumours. Dopamine antagonist and serotonin antagonist drugs (cyproheptadine) have a limited use in the treatment of ACTH-secreting tumours.

Treatment of the individual pituitary tumour depends upon the type involved.

1. *Prolactinomas.* A major development has been the demonstration that the dopamine agonist drug, bromocriptine, can shrink macroprolactinomas (Fig. 5.5), even if there has been extension above the sella compressing visual pathways. Treatment with this drug is an alternative to neurosurgery but special care must be taken in monitoring response to therapy. Cystic tumours are less likely to respond to medical treatment despite restoration of normal plasma prolactin levels. Once the tumour has been shrunk to within the confines of the pituitary fossa, external pituitary irradiation can be given to prevent recurrence. Bromocriptine therapy should be continued for a further 3 months whilst radiotherapy is taking effect. If bromocriptine is being used to restore fertility, patients are advised to discontinue therapy as soon as

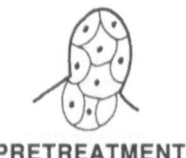
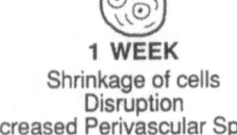
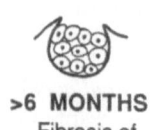

PRETREATMENT

1 WEEK
Shrinkage of cells
Disruption
Increased Perivascular Spaces

>6 MONTHS
Fibrosis of
Perivascular spaces

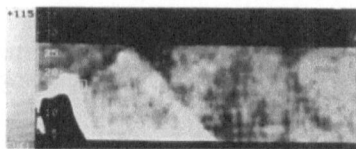
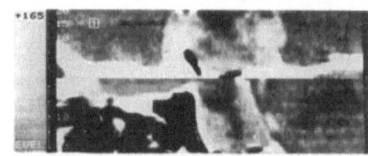

Fig. 5.5. Shrinkage of a macroprolactinoma with dopamine agonist treatment.

pregnancy is confirmed. However there is a significant risk (35%) of tumour expansion during pregnancy (Fig. 5.6). This risk appears to be minimised if the tumour is treated with external pituitary irradiation. Alternatively, an expectant policy may be justifiable with monthly assessment of visual fields and plasma prolactin concentrations. Elevation of plasma prolactin concentrations above the expected range for the stage of pregnancy, or symptoms suggesting tumour enlargement, are an immediate indication to restart bromocriptine treatment. Transsphenoidal neurosurgery is an alternative method of treating macroprolactinomas. Whilst surgical decompression will result in improved vision in 70% of cases, only 30% can expect a cure of their hyperprolactinaemia and this recurs in 80% by 3 years.

In patients with a microprolactinoma dopamine agonist therapy may therefore be the treatment of choice to deal with the symptoms of galactorrhoea and infertility. The risk of microprolactinoma expansion during pregnancy is less than 5% but monthly follow-up throughout pregnancy is advisable (Fig. 5.6). Transsphenoidal microsurgery is an alternative. In the short term, 85% of patients with a microprolactinoma can expect a cure (normoprolactinaemia) but in some centres up to 60% have relapsed in follow-up over 8 years. Patients with a microprolactinoma who are asymptomatic and do not wish fertility do not necessarily require treatment. One concern in not treating young patients with hyperprolactinaemia is that premature osteoporosis may result from prolactin-induced hypogonado-trophic hypogonadism.

2. *Growth-hormone-secreting tumours.* At present, transsphenoidal microsurgery and conventional pituitary irradiation appear to be the most effective, least damaging and most readily available forms of treatment for acromegaly. Transsphenoidal microsurgery is the treatment of choice, achieving a rapid reduction in hGH secretion with preservation of normal anterior pituitary

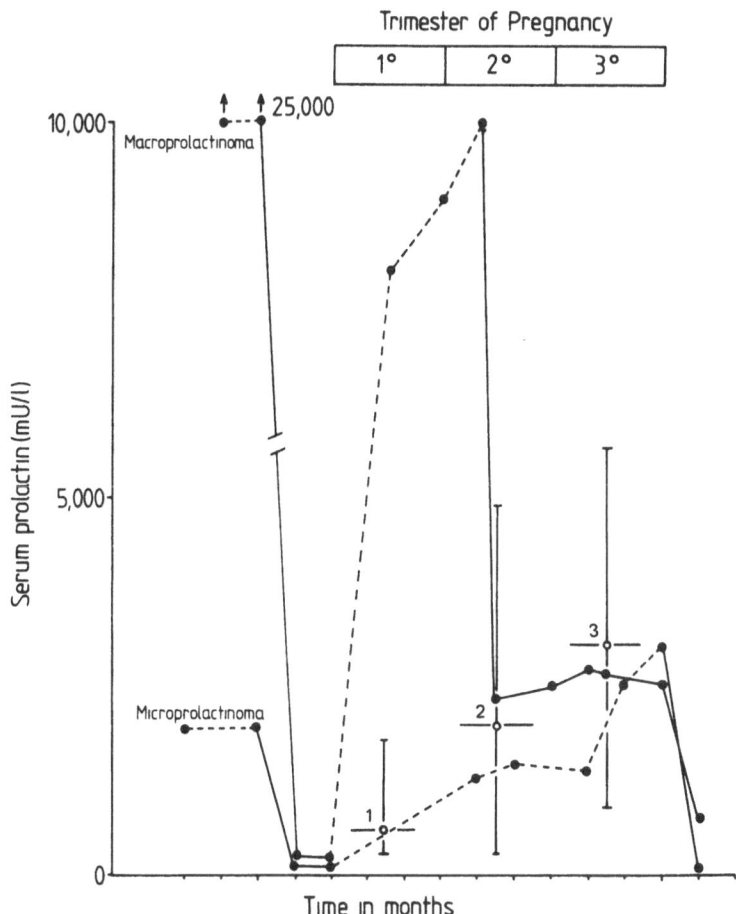

Fig. 5.6. Prolactin response to bromocriptine therapy and pregnancy in two patients, one with a microprolactinoma and the other with a macroprolactinoma. In the patient with a microprolactinoma, pregnancy was uneventful but in the patient with macroprolactinoma, drug withdrawal (– – –) and pregnancy stimulated prolactin secretion in excess of that expected for the first and second trimesters of pregnancy (*points 1 and 2*). The patient suffered severe headaches. However, reintroduction of bromocriptine (———) resulted in lowering of prolactin levels.

function in the majority of patients. A plasma hGH level of <10 mU/l can be achieved in 90% of patients with hGH-secreting microadenomas and in 60% of those with macroadenomas without visual field defects, but results are less favourable (30%) when macroadenomas are complicated by visual field defects. Long-term results of transsphenoidal surgery for hGH-secreting tumours are not yet available but if the postoperative plasma hGH level is

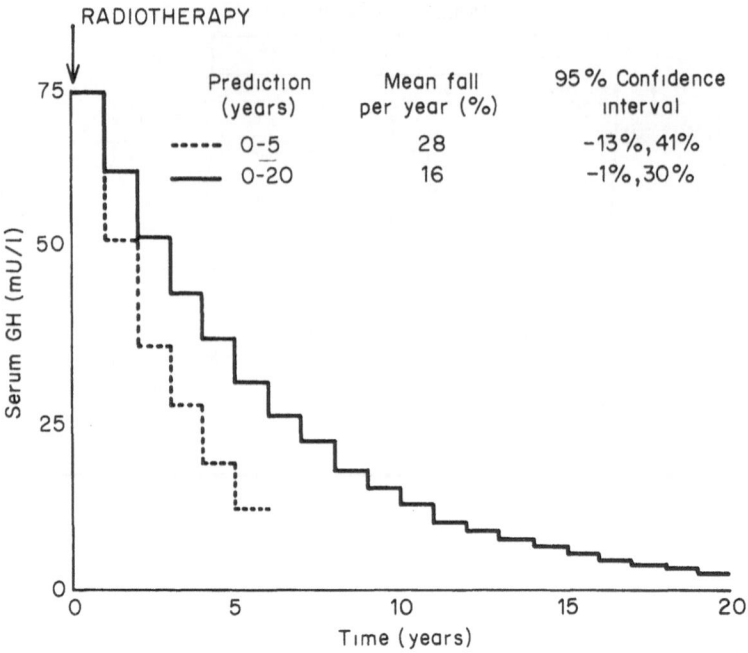

Fig. 5.7. The GH response to external pituitary irradiation (*arrow*) in patients with acromegaly.

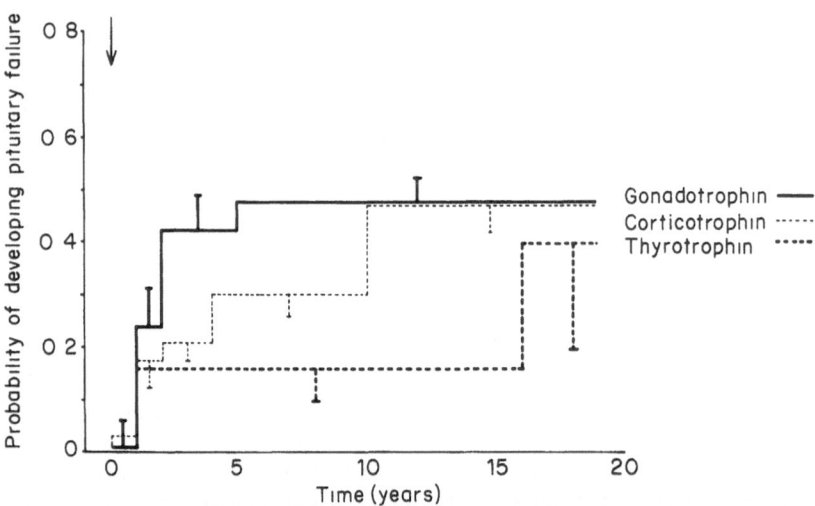

Fig. 5.8. The probability of developing anterior pituitary failure following external pituitary irradiation (*arrow*) increases with time.

raised, external irradiation is advised. Patients with normal levels should be carefully monitored for recurrence. Where external pituitary irradiation has been employed as the sole treatment, 45% of patients achieve a plasma hGH level of <10 mU/l by 5 years and 60% by 10 years (Fig. 5.7). However, there is also the complication of progressive anterior pituitary failure involving impaired gonadotrophin secretion in 50%, impaired ACTH secretion in 40% and impaired TSH secretion in 15% by 10 years (Fig. 5.8). Treatment with bromocriptine is only indicated as an adjunct to external pituitary irradiation in order to suppress plasma hGH levels whilst radiotherapy is taking effect.

3. *Corticotrophin-secreting tumours.* Transsphenoidal surgery is the treatment of choice and 80% of patients will be cured in the short term by an experienced neurosurgeon. Unfortunately very few long-term results are available. ACTH deficiency is common in the postoperative period resulting from suppression of normal corticotrophin-secreting cells that surround the tumour (Fig. 5.9). Recovery may take from 6 months to 2 years. During this period it is advisable to treat the patient with suboptimal doses of glucocorticoid (dexamethasone 0.5 mg daily) to provide sufficient replacement and permit recovery of the hypothalamic–pituitary–adrenal axis. If the plasma cortisol fails to decline to subnormal levels following the operation this may be used as an indication to re-explore the patient provided there is

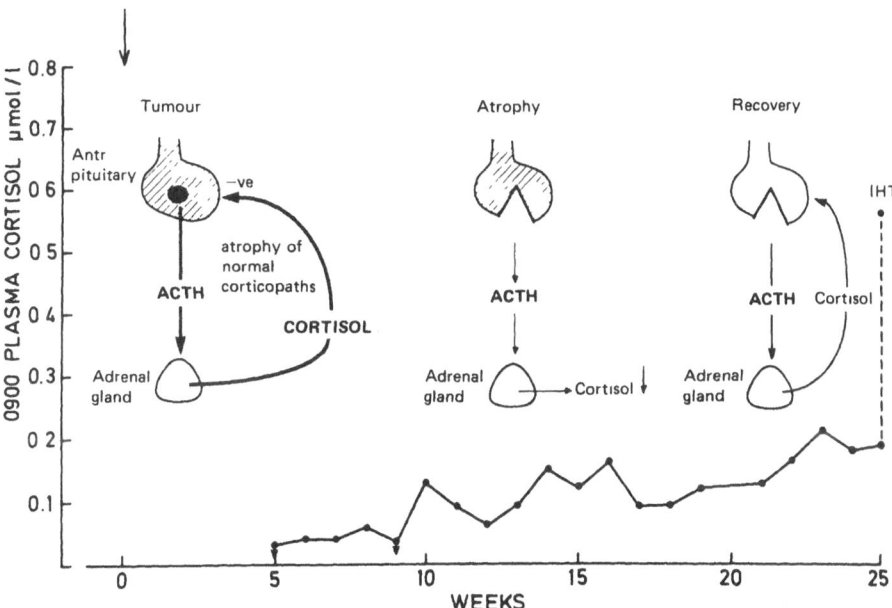

Fig. 5.9. The prolonged delay in recovery of cortisol secretion following transsphenoidal surgery for a corticotrophinoma (*arrow*). Six months elapse before full recovery of normal corticotrophin secretion is achieved in terms of a response to the insulin-induced hypoglycaemia test (IHT).

firm evidence that the pituitary is the cause of the Cushing's syndrome. Twenty per cent fail to respond to surgery. In 10% this reflects either the inability of the surgeon to find the tumour or the fact that the source of ACTH is ectopic from a tumour outside the pituitary gland. In 10% there is diffuse hyperplasia. It has been suggested that some corticotrophinomas originate from the intermediate lobe and ACTH secretion may be responsive to dopamine agonist therapy. Bilateral adrenalectomy is reserved for those who fail to respond to neurosurgery or those in whom an ectopic source cannot be localised. Bilateral adrenalectomy carries an operative mortality of 5%; hypercortisolaemia may recur from an adrenal remnant or accessory adrenal tissue despite an adequate operation. An expanding corticotrophinoma (Nelson's syndrome) develops in 20%–45% of patients unless the pituitary is irradiated at the time of adrenalectomy. External pituitary irradiation has been employed as primary treatment but requires concurrent medical treatment with metyrapone until the patient is cured, which only occurs in 20% of adults. It is, however, very effective for children with Cushing's disease.

4. *Non-functioning pituitary adenomas.* Management of these tumours involves replacing target hormones that have failed as a result of trophic hormone insufficiency and local treatment with surgery or radiotherapy when there is involvement of the optic pathways. In 15%, vision returns to normal; there is improvement in 70% and no change in 15%. If there is no suprasellar extension of the tumour, a conservative policy is often justified as these tumours are slow growing.

THE POSTERIOR PITUITARY

The hypothalamus synthesises arginine vasopressin as part of a large precursor molecule which is stored in neurosecretory granules and then migrates along axonal pathways to the posterior pituitary. Secretion of vasopressin into the systemic circulation is mainly determined by changes in plasma osmolality (Fig. 5.10). Vasopressin is suppressed by plasma osmolalities of less than 280 mosmol/kg and is secreted in direct relation to the plasma osmolality over the range 280–295 mosmol/kg. Thirst is experienced at a plasma osmolality of 300 mosmol/kg so that osmotic stimulation of vasopressin release and thirst maintain a plasma osmolality of 280–295 mosmol/kg in normal individuals. Pressure receptors in the left atrium of the heart play a minor role in vasopressin release under normal conditions but a more important role when there is a large fall in blood pressure. The kidney is the main target organ for the action of vasopressin, rendering the collecting tubules permeable to the passage of solute-free water from the hypotonic

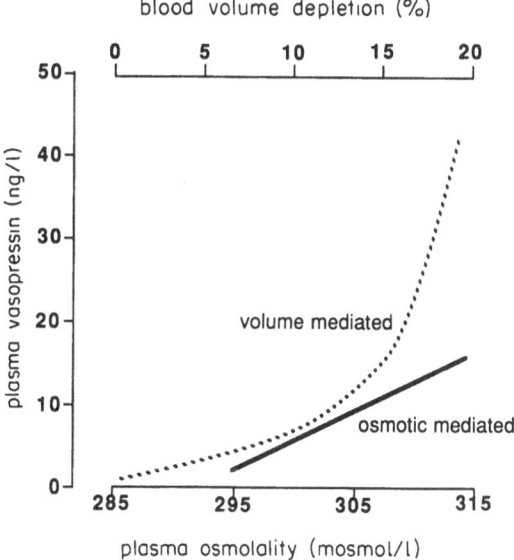

blood volume depletion (%)

Fig. 5.10. Osmotic-mediated and volume-mediated control of vasopressin release.

luminal fluid into the hypertonic interstitial renal medulla. This results in the formation of concentrated urine. In the absence of vasopressin the collecting tubule is impermeable to the passage of solute-free water which is passed as hypotonic urine.

Vasopressin Insufficiency

Diagnosis

Polyuria and polydypsia result from a deficiency of vasopressin (diabetes insipidus).

1. *Cranial causes* include pituitary tumours (25%), cranial surgery (20%), granulomas, infections, trauma (16%), metastases, infarction and, rarely, familial (dominant, recessive or associated with diabetes mellitus, optic atrophy and deafness: DIDMOAD syndrome). In a large number of cases (30%) the cause of cranial diabetes insipidus is unknown but may be related to an autoimmune hypophysitis.

2. *Nephrogenic causes* include hypercalcaemia, hypokalaemia, drugs (lithium and demethylchlortetracycline), solute excess (glycosuria), renal tract

obstruction, chronic renal diseases and a familial sex-linked recessive disorder.

3. *Compulsive water drinking* will suppress vasopressin secretion and cause nephrogenic diabetes insipidus by decreasing the tonicity of the interstitial renal medulla. Even if vasopressin is given to the patient, maximally concentrated urine cannot be formed because the osmotic gradient across the collecting tubule is reduced. With cranial and nephrogenic diabetes insipidus plasma osmolality is high and urine osmolality low whereas in compulsive water drinking both plasma and urine osmolalities are low. Urine output is in the order of 3–15 litres per day with cranial causes and responds to the administration of vasopressin. Nephrogenic causes are characterised by vasopressin-resistant polyuria. Observation of plasma and urine osmolality in response to water deprivation with subsequent administration of vasopressin is often required when the cause is in doubt (Fig. 5.11). It may be difficult to differentiate compulsive water drinking from nephrogenic diabetes insipidus.

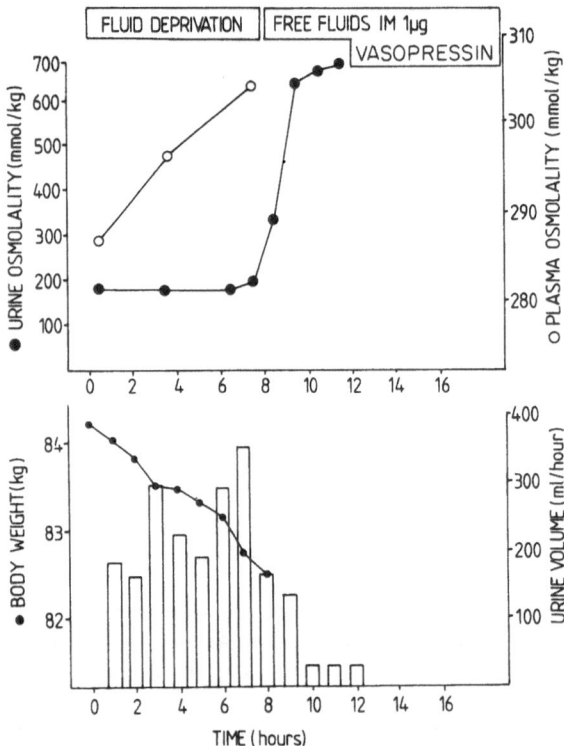

Fig. 5.11. Cranial diabetes during a period of water deprivation. Despite a progressive rise in plasma osmolality (300 mosmol/l) there is continued flow of dilute urine (200 mosmol/l). The patient subsequently responds to the exogenous administration of vasopressin.

Treatment

Cranial diabetes insipidus may require no specific treatment if it is mild with a urine output of only 3–4 litres per day, provided the patient is conscious and has an adequate thirst response. If it is more severe the patient should be treated with desmopressin, a long-acting synthetic vasopressin analogue with little pressor activity. Usually 10–20 μg is given by the nasal route or 1–2 μg intramuscularly twice daily. Care must be taken to avoid water intoxication. It is important to realise that cranial diabetes following trauma and neurosurgery may be transient, lasting from several days to 1 year. The need for antidiuretic therapy should therefore be reassessed in these patients periodically. The need for permanent treatment is usual with a high pituitary stalk lesion.

Nephrogenic diabetes insipidus is difficult to treat. However, thiazide diuretics, indomethacin and a low solute intake may be of help.

Compulsive water drinking usually responds to water restriction and treatment of any associated psychiatric disturbance.

Vasopressin Excess

The syndrome of inappropriate antidiuresis is one of the causes of dilutional hyponatraemia.

Diagnosis

The main features include hyponatraemia with appropriately low plasma osmolality, urine osmolality greater than that of plasma and persistent urinary sodium excretion in the absence of renal disease, adrenal disease, hypotension or volume depletion. Many conditions have been associated with inappropriate vasopressin secretion, namely various cancers including small cell carcinoma of the lung; neurological disorders including intracranial haemorrhage, head injury, tumours and infections; chest disorders including infections; hypothyroidism; and drugs. Drugs implicated in this syndrome are chlorpropamide, clofibrate, thiazides, phenothiazines, tricyclic antidepressants and some chemotherapeutic agents.

Treatment

If possible, hyponatraemia should be corrected by treatment of the underlying cause. The fluid intake should be restricted to 0.5–1 litre per day. For chronic hyponatraemia demeclocycline, up to 1.2 g daily, may be given in divided doses. It acts by inhibiting the action of vasopressin on the kidney causing a reversible nephrogenic diabetes insipidus. It is important to know that this drug may cause a photosensitive dermatitis.

6 Parathyroid Glands, Calcium and Bone Metabolism

The major organs involved in calcium homeostasis are the intestine, kidneys and bone. Parathyroid hormone (PTH), vitamin D_3 and, possibly, calcitonin act to maintain ionised plasma calcium levels within the normal range (Fig. 6.1).

Calcium is transported in the blood bound to albumin but only the free ionised fraction is biologically active, regulating the secretion of PTH. PTH in turn regulates the level of free calcium in the blood by its actions on bone, kidney and vitamin D metabolism. Routine plasma calcium estimations measure total plasma calcium and the value obtained should be interpreted in the light of the prevailing plasma albumin level. Alkalosis decreases ionised calcium, and symptomatic hypocalcaemia may be a feature of hyperventilation. For each gram of albumin above or below a nominal mean of 42 g/l, 0.02 mmol/l of calcium is respectively subtracted or added to the measured plasma calcium. Using this correction, the upper limit of corrected plasma calcium is 2.6 mmol/l, but this correction should be interpreted with caution in the presence of wide deviations in plasma protein concentrations. The daily intake of calcium is around 25 mmol but only 7.5 mmol is absorbed by the intestine into the plasma calcium pool and the remainder is excreted in the faeces. The plasma pool receives a further contribution of 1.25 mmol from bone resorption but balance is maintained with losses of 1.25 mmol to bone formation, 3.75 mmol to intestinal secretion (total faecal output 21.25 mmol) and 3.75 mmol in urinary excretion. In the absence of an adequate dietary intake of calcium, plasma calcium levels are maintained at the expense of bone.

The three major cell types of bone are osteoblasts, osteocytes and osteoclasts. Osteoblasts are responsible for the synthesis of the extracellular bone matrix, secretion of alkaline phosphatase (a marker of osteoblastic activity) and priming of its subsequent mineralisation. Osteocytes are derived from osteoblasts and lie within mineralised bone arranged in concentric layers. Osteoclasts decalcify and digest the protein matrix of bone, liberating calcium and hydroxyproline (a marker of osteoclastic activity).

PTH and vitamin D_3 stimulate osteoclastic bone resorption whereas calcitonin and oestrogens are inhibitory. In the kidney, PTH enhances

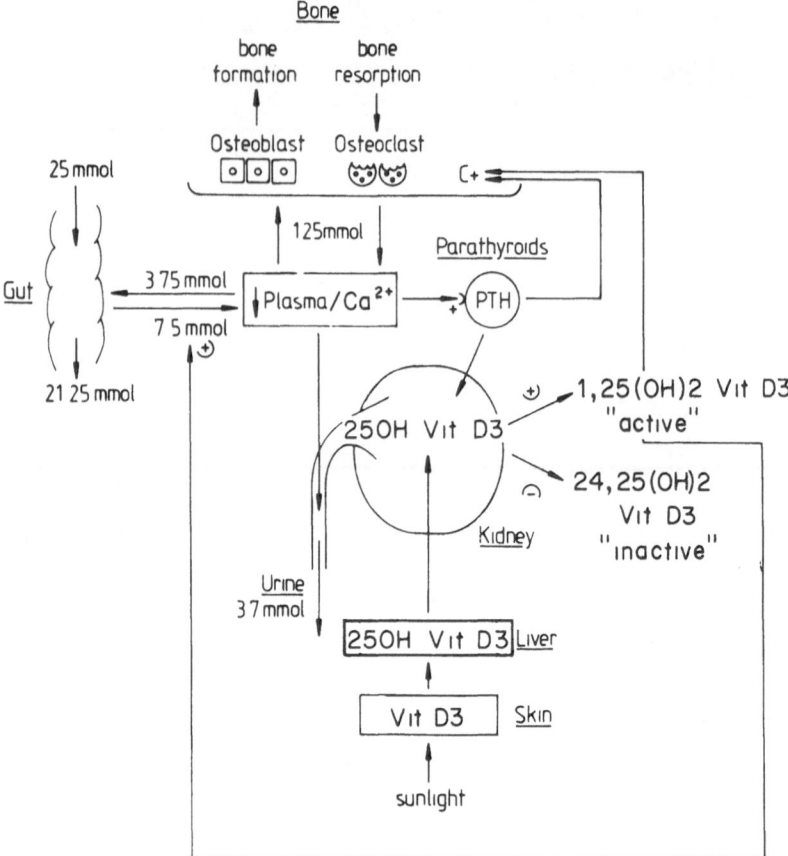

Fig. 6.1. Hormonal regulation of plasma calcium concentrations.

calcium reabsorption in the ascending loop and distal tubules and inhibits proximal tubular reabsorption of phosphate leading to hypercalcaemia and hypophosphataemia. These actions are mediated by the adenyl cyclase system and there is a parallel increased urinary excretion of sodium, potassium and bicarbonate. Urinary excretion of cyclic AMP can be used as an index of PTH activity. Vitamin D_3 metabolism is activated by PTH to promote the intestinal absorption of calcium.

The major source of vitamin D_3 is the skin following the photoconversion of 7-dehydrocholesterol to vitamin D_3. Increased skin pigmentation can greatly reduce the synthesis of vitamin D_3. Under normal circumstances the dietary contribution to vitamin D_3 stores is insignificant. Vitamin D_3 is removed from the skin to the general circulation by a transport protein in the blood. It is then hydroxylated by the liver to 25OH vitamin D_3 and again in the kidney to either biologically active $1,25(OH)_2$ vitamin D_3 or inactive $24,25(OH)_2$ vitamin D_3. PTH, hypocalcaemia and hypophosphataemia preferentially stimulate formation of active $1,25(OH)_2$ vitamin D_3 and inhibit formation of the inactive $24,25(OH)_2$ metabolite. $1,25(OH)_2$ Vitamin D_3 promotes the absorption of calcium and phosphate from the gut, promotes bone resorption and acts on the kidney to increase calcium and phosphate reabsorption.

Hypocalcaemia

Decreased ionised calcium levels in the plasma cause increased neuroexcitability. Symptoms of hypocalcaemia include numbness and tingling in the extremities or around the mouth, muscle cramps and eventually carpo-pedal spasm. Chvostek's and Trousseau's signs are positive. However, these symptoms and signs may also be seen in cases of hypokalaemia and hypomagnesaemia. Prolonged hypocalcaemia may result in cataracts.

Diagnosis

Hypocalcaemia with Low Plasma PTH Levels

Hypocalcaemia and hyperphosphataemia are the features of hypoparathyroidism.

1. *Postoperative hypoparathyroidism* is the commonest cause and occurs following thyroid surgery, parathyroid surgery and other neck operations.

2. *Autoimmune hypoparathyroidism* is a rare disorder associated with autoimmune adrenalitis (Addison's disease), atrophic gastritis (pernicious anaemia), diabetes mellitus and thyroid disease. Other clinical features of this disorder include epilepsy, mental retardation and papilloedema with intracerebral calcification of the basal ganglia. Dentition is poor, nails are dystrophic and become infected with candida; skin is dry and scaly with sparse hair growth.

3. *Neonatal hypocalcaemia* may occur transiently in children of mothers with hyperparathyroidism; fetal parathyroid glands are presumably suppressed by maternal hypercalcaemia. (Hypocalcaemia is also seen in the neonatal period as a result of feeding infants with phosphate-rich foods such as cow's milk.)

4. *Magnesium deficiency* is an important cause of hypocalcaemia which can be readily reversed by the administration of magnesium supplements alone. Conditions associated with magnesium deficiency are malabsorption, alcoholism and prolonged parenteral feeding. Hypomagnesaemia causes suppression

of the parathyroid glands and skeletal and renal resistance to the action of PTH.

5. *Acute pancreatitis* may be accompanied by hypoalbuminaemia and low plasma calcium levels. Low ionised plasma calcium levels are attributed to sequestration of calcium in abdominal deposits of necrotic fat. However there also appears to be impaired secretion of PTH, preventing maintenance of normal plasma calcium levels. Associated hypomagnesaemia will exacerbate the problem.

Hypocalcaemia with Raised Plasma PTH Levels

Secondary hyperparathyroidism is a normal physiological response to hypocalcaemia.

1. *Osteomalacia and rickets* may require bone biopsy for definitive diagnosis. Less than 60% of osteoid surfaces have calcification fronts and mineralisation rate is reduced, whereas osteoid seam thickness, osteoid surfaces and bone occupied by osteoid are increased. Children present with growth failure and swelling and deformity at sites of maximal bone growth, the site depending on the stage of development. Adults present with bone pain and a proximal myopathy. Routine biochemistry reveals hypocalcaemia and hypophosphataemia in 60% of cases, and 90% have elevated plasma alkaline phosphatase levels. Secondary hyperparathyroidism is evidenced by raised plasma PTH levels. Plasma 25OH vitamin D_3 is reduced in over 60% of patients. The causes are often complex.

a) Vitamin D_3 deficiency can be due to environmental factors or intestinal disease. In the early part of this century the prevalence of rickets was high in all the major cities of northern Europe where sunlight exposure was deficient because of industrial pollution, latitude and poor housing. With improved public health measures the disease virtually disappeared only to reappear in the immigrant Asian community whose skin and traditional habits in diet and dress are inappropriate for the northern latitude of the UK. Osteomalacia is also common in the elderly because of inadequate exposure to sunlight due to immobility in a population whose dietary intake is poor. However, in the presence of adequate sunlight dietary sources are of minor importance and the association of vitamin D_3 deficiency with intestinal diseases, particularly malabsorption syndromes, can be adequately explained by interference with the enterohepatic circulation.

b) Defective synthesis of 25OH vitamin D_3 could theoretically occur in patients with liver disease, but even in severe failure 25-hydroxylation is adequate to meet body requirements. Anticonvulsant and antituberculous drugs are said to interfere with hepatic metabolism of vitamin D_3 to explain the well-recognised association of osteomalacia with the chronic ingestion of these drugs. It is more likely that osteomalacia results from inadequate exposure to sunlight as in environmental osteomalacia.

c) Defective $1,25(OH)_2$ vitamin D_3 synthesis occurs in chronic renal failure and rarely as a hereditary defect in renal 1α-hydroxylase. In chronic renal disease osteomalacia may present 2–3 years after the onset of renal failure. Biochemically a wide spectrum of abnormalities is present due to the combined effect of secondary hyperparathyroidism, osteomalacia and renal failure. Plasma calcium estimations may be low, normal or even high where tertiary hyperparathyroidism has developed. Plasma phosphate is often elevated due to renal failure and plasma PTH levels are raised to greater levels than would be expected because of impaired excretion. Plasma alkaline phosphatase is elevated and plasma $1,25(OH)_2$ vitamin D_3 levels are low but 25OH vitamin D_3 levels may be normal depending on the exposure to sunlight. The severity of osteomalacia correlates with the severity of the acidosis. The administration of aluminium hydroxide to reduce plasma phosphate levels in an attempt to reduce secondary hyperparathyroidism leads to phosphate depletion and exacerbates osteomalacia. Following maintenance haemodialysis the situation becomes more complex with an increased incidence of osteomalacia due to a combination of renal failure, phosphate depletion and aluminium toxicity. The osteomalacia may respond to appropriate vitamin D therapy but ectopic calcification may occur with the rise in plasma calcium. Usually hyperparathyroidism fails to resolve until treated surgically. Renal transplantation generally improves renal bone disease and hyperparathyroidism but parathyroid surgery is still required in 20% of cases.

2. *Pseudohypoparathyroidism* has all the features of hypoparathyroidism with hypocalcaemia, hyperphosphataemia and decreased urinary cyclic AMP excretion with hypophosphaturia. However, plasma PTH levels are elevated and a defect in coupling of the renal PTH receptor to the adenyl cyclase system has been demonstrated. Children present before the age of 8 years and over 50% are mentally retarded. In addition to the classical features of hypocalcaemia there are associated skeletal abnormalities such as a short, thickset habitus with a round face and short neck. Short fourth and fifth metacarpals are characteristic and basal ganglia calcification is seen in 50% of cases.

Treatment

Severe acute hypocalcaemia with symptoms of tetany may occur following neck surgery, with autoimmune hypoparathyroidism and pseudohypopara-thyroidism and with osteomalacia associated with renal or gastrointestinal diseases. It should be treated with intravenous calcium gluconate. Initially 10 ml of 10% calcium gluconate (2.25 mmol) is given followed by an infusion of 1.7 ml/kg of 10% calcium gluconate in either saline or glucose 5% over a 4-hour period. If magnesium deficiency is also present this should be corrected by the intravenous administration of magnesium chloride 0.25 mmol/kg in either saline or glucose 5% over a 4-hour period. Following acute treatment and for less severe cases of hypocalcaemia oral treatment may be started with oral calcium in the form of effervescent calcium tablets, 10 mmol 8-hourly. If oral magnesium is required, magnesium gluconate, 1 mmol/kg daily, can be given in divided doses (each sachet contains 10 mmol). Vitamin D should also be started (see below) and oral calcium withdrawn as soon as the plasma calcium level reaches the normal range.

Chronic hypocalcaemia is treated by the administration of "high dose" vitamin D_3 (calciferol) or one of its metabolites. The pharmacological and biological half-life of calciferol is long; it takes 4–8 weeks to restore normocalcaemia, 4–10 weeks to reach maximum effect and its effect persists for 6–18 weeks following withdrawal. In contrast, 1α-OH vitamin D_3 (alphacalcidol) has a much more rapid biological effect, restoring normocalcaemia within 1 week; its effect persists for only 1 week following withdrawal, permitting greater flexibility in manipulation of the dosage. The dose of calciferol is 1.25–2.5 mg daily and on these doses 24% will achieve normocalcaemia, but 70% will have episodes of hypocalcaemia and 6% hypercalcaemia. The dose of alphacalcidol is 1–3 μg daily and 40% will achieve normocalcaemia but 55% will have hypocalcaemic episodes and 5% hypercalcaemia.

Osteomalacia that is environmental or drug induced will respond completely to a course of ultraviolet irradiation or "low-dose" vitamin D_3 therapy. In these cases vitamin D_3 should be prescribed as "calcium with vitamin D tablets" containing calciferol 12.5 μg and calcium 2 mmol. Osteomalacia associated with malabsorption requires either "high-dose" vitamin D_3 therapy in the form of intramuscular calciferol 250–2500 μg per week or "high doses" of the well-absorbed hydroxylated metabolites such as alphacalcidol 2–4 μg daily. The mineralisation defect of renal osteodystrophy resolves on "high-dose" therapy with alphacalcidol 1μg daily.

Hypercalcaemia

The commonest symptoms of hypercalcaemia are malaise, depression, nausea, vomiting, constipation and polyuria and polydypsia due to nephrogenic diabetes insipidus. One of the commonest causes of hypercalcaemia is primary hyperparathyroidism which in addition to hypercalcaemia causes a proximal renal tubular acidosis with inhibition of tubular phosphate reabsorption, resulting in a hyperchloraemic acidosis, and hypophosphataemia and increased excretion of phosphate and cyclic AMP in the urine. In non-parathyroid hypercalcaemia the converse is true.

Whilst the two groups of hypercalcaemic patients have certain biochemical differences there is considerable overlap, posing difficulties in the diagnosis of the individual case. The most useful single test should be the measurement of plasma PTH, with elevated levels in hyperparathyroidism and suppressed values in non-parathyroid cases. Unfortunately many assays cannot do this. Biological activity of PTH resides in the N-terminal region whereas many of the fragments detected in the circulation are derived from the mid-region or C-terminal region. With N-terminal assays 80% of patients with hyperparathyroidism have elevated levels of PTH whereas PTH detected by C-terminal assay is elevated in all cases. If a satisfactory assay for PTH is unavailable a steroid suppression test should be performed. Plasma calcium is estimated before and after the administration of oral hydrocortisone 40 mg 8-hourly for 10 days. A fall in the corrected fasting plasma calcium of more than 0.25 mmol/l indicates adequate suppression. Ninety-eight per cent of patients with primary hyperparathyroidism fail to suppress in response to steroid administration but this falls to 65% if there is associated bone involvement. Ninety-four per cent of patients with non-parathryoid hypercalcaemia suppress following hydrocortisone.

Diagnosis

Hypercalcaemia with Suppressed Plasma PTH Levels

This is caused by a wide variety of conditions.

1. *Malignancies* account for 40% of cases of hypercalcaemia and are commonly carcinomas of lung and breast. In most patients with malignant hypercalcaemia there is clinical evidence of obvious malignant disease. In many patients there are no bone metastases and the tumour-induced hypercalcaemia is caused by humoral factors produced by the tumour. These include transforming growth factors, prostaglandins, osteoclast-activating factor and only rarely PTH.

2. *Vitamin D poisoning* is the third commonest cause of hypercalcaemia. This can occur when the correct dose is prescribed for the appropriate condition, but in 25% of cases vitamin D poisoning results from inappropriate indications or the use of "high-dose" vitamin D therapy where "low doses" are indicated.

3. Hypercalcaemia is a recognised complication of *hyperthyroidism* in 17% of cases and is thought to be due to a direct action of thyroid hormones on bone turnover increasing bone resorption. This leads to hypercalcaemia and suppression of plasma PTH levels.

4. Less than 1% of patients with *sarcoidosis* develop hypercalcaemia, often in the summer months, associated with abnormal $1,25(OH)_2$ vitamin D_3 levels. Overproduction of $1,25(OH)_2$ vitamin D_3 by the sarcoid tissue appears to be responsible for hypercalcaemia rather than increased sensitivity to normal vitamin D_3 levels. A similar mechanism has been postulated in tuberculosis.

5. *The milk-alkali syndrome* is a rare condition associated with excessive ingestion of calcium in the form of milk and an excessive amount of soluble alkali. It is now uncommon following the introduction of non-absorbable alkalis.

Hypercalcaemia with Raised Plasma PTH Levels

1. *Primary hyperparathyroidism* has a prevalence of 1–3 per 1000 and accounts for 50% of cases of hypercalcaemia. It is rarely associated with MEN types 1 and 2 (see section on adrenal medulla). Approximately 30% of patients present with bone disease, 30% with renal calculi and 10% with mixed presentations. However, 30% are asymptomatic and are detected by routine biochemical analysis. Patients with bone disease are older, have larger parathyroid glands, higher plasma PTH levels, lower plasma 25OH vitamin D_3 levels and lower urinary calcium excretion than those with renal involvement. The simplest explanation of these findings is that patients with hyperparathyroidism develop bone disease if they have lower vitamin D_3 stores (in general vitamin D_3 levels are increased in hyperparathyroidism) but if these stores are adequate, increased intestinal absorption of calcium leads to hypercalciuria, renal calculi and a renal presentation. Bone disease is manifested by an elevated plasma alkaline phosphatase in 30%, osteopenia in 25%, classical radiological features of subperiosteal erosions in 13% and by osteitis fibrosa cystica in 4%. The renal tract should be investigated radiologically in all patients with proven hyperparathyroidism. Other features include hypertension, proximal myopathy, chondrocalcinosis and peptic ulceration due to calcium-mediated stimulation of gastrin secretion. Only some of these features are reversible following restoration of normal plasma calcium levels. Hypertension usually persists.

2. *Familial hypocalciuric hypercalcaemia* is a familial syndrome accounting for up to 10% of failed neck explorations for hyperparathyroidism. The cardinal features are hypercalcaemia associated with hypocalciuria (<5 mmol/day), hypermagnesaemia and a pattern of inheritance compatible with an autosomal dominant trait with partial penetrance. Plasma PTH concentrations and stigmata of hyperparathyroidism in terms of a proximal renal tubular acidosis, inhibition of tubular phosphate reabsorption and urinary excretion of cyclic AMP are intermediate between normal and hyperparathyroid individuals.

3. *Thiazide diuretics.* The mechanism is obscure but the majority of these patients appear to have underlying primary hyperparathyroidism, and elevated plasma calcium levels may respond to withdrawal of the drug.

4. *Tertiary hyperparathyroidism* is the development of autonomous parathyroid function in patients with longstanding secondary hyperparathyroidism (e.g. chronic renal failure).

Treatment

Severe acute hypercalcaemia should be treated with rehydration with intravenous physiological saline in a sufficient volume to achieve an adequate diuresis. Potassium replacement may be necessary as hypercalcaemic patients are hypokalaemic from renal tubular damage. A formal steroid suppression test (hydrocortisone 40 mg 8-hourly orally for 10 days) is valuable at this stage for therapeutic as well as diagnostic reasons. Following the steroid suppression test the physician should be in a better position to diagnose the underlying cause with additional information from plasma PTH levels, protein electrophoresis, urinary light chain excretion, chest radiology, skeletal radiology and skeletal scintigraphy if necessary. If symptomatic hypercalcaemia persists two additional lines of treatment may be considered:

1. Hypercalcaemia resulting from increased bone resorption can be blocked by the administration of salmon calcitonin 200 units 6-hourly by subcutaneous or intravenous injection. Calcitonin alone is only effective for 2 days following which "escape" occurs possibly due to down-regulation of bone calcitonin receptors. In combination with corticosteroids (prednisolone 60 mg daily in divided doses) it is much more effective, reducing plasma calcium levels for 4 days or more. Alternatively mithramycin 25 µg/kg given as an intravenous bolus causes a significant fall in plasma calcium in 24–36 hours. It cannot be given for more than a few days because of marrow toxicity. In the future, diphosphonates such as intravenous aminopropylidene diphosphonate 15 mg daily promise to be effective.

2. Plasma calcium levels can be acutely lowered as an emergency in patients with life-threatening hypercalcaemia by the intravenous administration of 25 mmol neutral phosphate buffer over 6 hours. Risks of this treatment include ectopic calcification, renal failure and sudden death. These complications are probably rare but indicate that intravenous phosphate should only be given when other methods have failed. Oral phosphate 5 g 8-hourly may be given much more safely but the dose may have to be lowered because of troublesome diarrhoea.

Less severe hypercalcaemia is best treated with oral rehydration.

Chronic hypercalcaemia is managed according to the underlying disorder.

The definitive treatment of hyperparathyroidism is surgical and this is indicated for symptomatic patients with bone or renal involvement. There is considerable debate as to the need for surgery in patients who are asymptomatic. However, when plasma calcium levels are in excess of 2.75 mmol/l patients should probably be referred for surgery whilst those with levels below this should be carefully monitored. If plasma calcium levels do not change over a 3-month period it is reasonably safe to monitor the patient annually with plasma and urinary calcium estimations, plain abdominal radiology and tests of renal function. Any change in these parameters should lead to reconsideration of the need for definitive treatment. These guidelines are arbitrary and may be modified in the light of other factors such as the patient's age.

Preoperative localisation is probably unnecessary. Hyperparathyroidism is caused by a single adenoma in 90% of cases, diffuse hyperplasia in 9% and in 1% by a carcinoma. At surgery all four glands should be identified but if no abnormality is found and one of the glands is missing from its anatomical site, the neck, thyroid and thymus should be carefully examined. If the missing gland is not found, a thyroid lobectomy is performed on the missing side for a possible intrathyroidal gland and the operation concluded. Most mediastinal adenomas can be retrieved from the neck so that splitting of the sternum is not routinely necessary (1% of parathyroid operations). Hyperplasia may be suspected at operation because all four glands are easy to see; this may be primary or tertiary. Two operations are available in cases of hyperplasia: either removal of three and a half glands leaving a half behind or total parathyroidectomy with reimplantation of half a gland in the forearm. In the former the gland should be identified with a clip in case re-exploration is needed but it is obviously easier to operate on the forearm than the neck. However, long-term evaluation of forearm implantation is required as failure of PTH secretion by the implant has now been described even 2 years after surgery.

In the postoperative period temporary hypocalcaemia occurs in 20% of patients, particularly if there is bone involvement; patients who have bone involvement should therefore be commenced on oral alphacalcidol 1–2 μg daily starting the day before operation. Eleven per cent develop permanent hypoparathyroidism which can be treated with vitamin D or implantation of cryopreserved parathyroid tissue if this is made available at the time of operation. The majority of parathyroid explorations are successful, resulting in removal of the abnormal tissue and restoration of normal plasma calcium levels. A failed operation is often due to inexperience and the choice of a good surgeon and experienced pathologist is critical to the outcome. Before reoperation an attempt should be made to localise abnormal glands by venous sampling for PTH "hot spots" in the circulation in the neck and by ultrasound if high-resolution real-time equipment and experience are available.

Surgery is not recommended for those patients with familial hypocalciuric hypercalcaemia as over 50% remain hypercalcaemic after operation and the condition is essentially benign.

Osteoporosis

Osteopenia is the term used to describe bones that appear "thin" on routine radiographs. It is not radiographically possible to distinguish between osteoporosis and osteomalacia on the basis of bone density alone; this difference is made on histological and biochemical grounds. In osteomalacia there is a reduction in bone mineral content but bone mass is normal, whereas in osteoporosis the reduction in bone mineral content is secondary to the reduction in bone mass (Fig. 6.2). Osteoporosis is a major public health problem being a major risk factor for fractures of wrist, spine and neck of femur. The cumulative prevalence of these three fractures in women is respectively 5, 2.5 and 0.4% by the age of 60, increasing to 15, 7.5 and 6% by the age of 80. The increase in fracture rates corresponds to an age-related loss

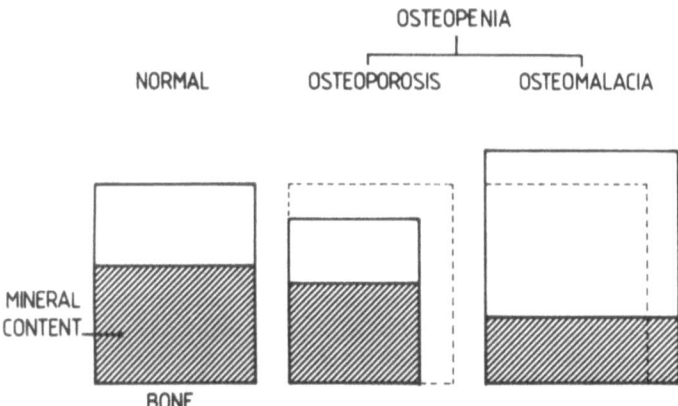

Fig. 6.2. The volume of anatomical bone in osteoporosis, osteomalacia and normal bone.

of bone mass, resulting in a higher proportion of the population with a bone mass below the critical threshold for fracture (Fig. 6.3).

Diagnosis

Simple osteoporosis is the natural loss of bone mass that occurs with age. Approximately 15% of the skeleton is lost between the ages of 40 and 80; trabecular bone (vertebrae) is lost progressively over this period whereas loss of cortical bone (wrist and predominantly femur) is maximal between 40 and 60 and is self-limiting thereafter.

Osteoporosis affects women more than men. In women the reduction in bone mass is a result of increased bone resorption associated with oestrogen

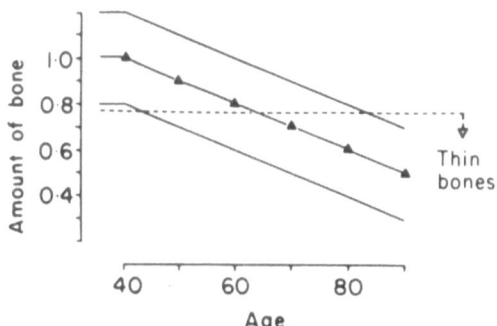

Fig. 6.3. Declining volume of anatomical bone with age increases the proportion of the population at risk of falling below the threshold at which spontaneous bone fractures occur.

deficiency following the menopause. Increased bone resorption leads to higher plasma calcium levels, increased urinary calcium excretion and subsequent suppression of PTH secretion. Consequently, formation of $1,25(OH)_2$ vitamin D_3 is reduced, decreasing absorption of calcium from the gut. The situation of increased bone resorption with increased urinary calcium loss is therefore aggravated by impaired absorption of calcium. The administration of oestrogens can reverse this situation. In men, osteoporosis results from reduced bone formation as testosterone secretion declines with increasing age.

Accelerated osteoporosis occurs when the rate of loss of bone exceeds the normal rate. Risk factors in the development of accelerated osteoporosis include hyperthyroidism, excessive glucocorticoid secretion or administration, acromegaly, malabsorption syndromes, cigarette smoking, liver disease, diabetes mellitus and diet. Occasionally, accelerated osteoporosis occurs in patients in whom none of these risk factors can be identified (idiopathic osteoporosis).

Treatment

Acute back pain is the most serious consequence for the patient following a vertebral crush fracture. Acute episodes require 2–3 weeks bed rest with adequate analgesia, followed by gradual mobilisation. A corset is often helpful and the patient should be taught extension exercises of the spine to recover the normal lumbar lordosis. This advice is usually given by a skilled physiotherapist. Swimming is a form of exercise that should be encouraged.

Chronic back pain related to old fracture sites will partially respond to medical therapy. The mainstay of current medical treatment is to prevent further loss of bone mass.

1. *Sex steroids* are used to inhibit bone resorption. In women below 50 in whom oestrogens are not contraindicated, ethinyl oestradiol is administered in doses of 10–20 μg daily for 3 weeks out of 4. Medroxyprogesterone acetate 5 mg daily is given in the 3rd week to prevent the risk of endometrial carcinoma induced by the unopposed action of oestrogens. However it is difficult to know for how long therapy should be continued. On the available evidence treatment should be given for a minimum of 5 years. The patient should be carefully monitored and if the rate of bone loss increases, oestrogen therapy may have to be reintroduced. In men, testosterone (testosterone esters: Sustanon) is given by intramuscular injection in a dose of 100 mg weekly.

2. *Oral calcium* is useful even in cases with normal calcium absorption because increased loss of calcium from the skeleton needs to be met by an increased dietary intake. Effervescent calcium may be given in doses of 30 mmol daily. When combined with oestrogen therapy, calcium reduces fracture rates to 25% of the pretreatment level although bone mass is only minimally increased. The addition of vitamin D to the regimen is of no further

benefit and is associated with a substantial incidence of hypercalcaemia or hypercalciuria.

The response of these regimens should be carefully monitored by estimation of plasma calcium levels at 3-month intervals and by height, lateral thoracolumbar spinal radiography and estimation of bone mass at yearly intervals. Current methods of estimation of bone mass include radiographic metacarpal morphometry, single or dual photon absorptiometry, computerised tomography and total body calcium by neutron activation analysis. Further treatment should be considered if there is no reduction in the rate of fracture, there is loss of height, deterioration radiographically or continued fall in bone mass. In these patients the addition of sodium fluoride in daily doses of 75 mg to the combination of calcium and oestrogen therapy can further reduce fracture rates to 15% of pretreatment levels. This treatment is associated with a significant increase in bone mass resulting from stimulation of bone formation without stimulation of bone resorption. The increase is predominantly in the trabecular bone of the axial skeleton whereas cortical bone mass is significantly decreased. Fluoride therapy should help protect against vertebral crush fractures but may increase fractures of the proximal femur.

Paget's Disease

The overall prevalence of Paget's disease is 3%–5%, increasing with age to affect 5% of women and 10% of men by the age of 80. Paget's disease is primarily a disorder of osteoclasts. In the active phase of this disease overactive osteoclasts resorb bone at a much greater rate than normal with increased urinary excretion of hydroxyproline. Electron microscopy has revealed that the ultrastructure of the osteoclast is compatible with a slow virus infection. Osteoblastic activity becomes secondarily increased with elevated plasma alkaline phosphatase levels. Bone turnover is increased 20 times. Cycles of bone destruction and new bone formation follow each other, resulting in disorderly deposition of bone that is mechanically less efficient and easily deformed. The activity of the osteoclast gradually declines whilst the osteoblast continues to lay down new bone at a rapid pace to cover the area previously resorbed. However, the bone formed is abnormal, lacking Haversian systems, and lamellar bone with irregular cement lines is the prominent component. Osteoblastic activity then declines.

Diagnosis

The majority of patients are asymptomatic and are discovered during a routine clinical, radiological or biochemical examination. The spine is involved in 50% of cases, skull 30%, pelvis 20%, femur 20%, tibia 10% and humerus 5%. More than one bone is affected in 75% of patients. Five per cent are symptomatic with local pain and deformity. Complications of Paget's disease include pathological fracture, osteoarthrosis, nerve compression, basilar invagination of the skull, hypercalcaemia with immobilisation, heart failure and sarcoma. Malignant change occurs in less than 1% and carries a poor prognosis with a 5-year survival of 5%.

Treatment

Patients should be assessed with estimation of urinary hydroxyproline excretion, plasma alkaline phosphatase and ^{99m}Tc bone scintigraphy. The majority of patients require no treatment, indications being pain and the development of complications:

1. *Calcitonin* directly inhibits osteoclastic bone resorption, producing an acute reduction in plasma calcium levels over 6–8 hours. It is most marked in those patients with an increased bone turnover rate. In the long term, plasma alkaline phosphatase levels and urinary hydroxyproline excretion fall to 50% of pretreatment values. Salmon calcitonin is recommended, being more potent than either porcine or human calcitonins, and is more resistant to renal metabolism than human calcitonin whereas porcine calcitonin is metabolised by the liver. However, 60% of patients receiving porcine and 30% receiving salmon calcitonins may develop antibodies which may be significant enough to interfere with therapy on rare occasions. Human calcitonin does not appear to be antigenic. Initially, salmon calcitonin 100 units daily is given by subcutaneous injection, reducing to 50–100 units three times a week after 1 month; treatment is continued for 1 year. Calcitonin can then be discontinued providing a maximum response has been achieved. Pain is reduced in 80%, fracture rates are reduced and neurological complications may be significantly improved in 75%. Treatment is associated with a reduction in the uptake of bone-seeking isotopes and improved bone structure. Bone mass is increased in association with increased bone mineralisation and decreased bone resorption. Side-effects are few but include mild nausea. Following withdrawal it takes approximately 6 months for plasma alkaline phosphatase levels and urinary hydroxyproline excretion to return to pretreatment values. However the longer the treatment period the greater is the delay in the rise in these parameters.

2. *Diphosphonates* inhibit bone resorption and mineralisation by binding to hydroxyapatite crystals and inhibiting their growth and dissolution. They are structural analogues of inorganic pyrophosphates in which the unstable phosphorus–oxygen bonds (P–O–P) are replaced by P–C–P bonds that are more resistant to degradation. Biopsies of treated patients show that overactive osteoclasts and osteoblasts are replaced by a more normal bone population in association with biochemical evidence of suppression of the active lesion. The main advantage of this group of drugs over calcitonin is that they may be administered by mouth. The main disadvantage of prolonged

administration is that the incidence of fractures and bone pain may increase and focal osteomalacia may develop on histology. Disodium etidronate administration in doses of 5 mg/kg daily over a 6-month period is optimal, producing symptomatic improvement and a 50% reduction in plasma alkaline phosphatase levels and urinary hydroxyproline excretion. After discontinuation 15% of patients require no further treatment for up to 5 years, 50% require repeated cycles of 6 months of disodium etidronate therapy alternating with 6 months or more of no therapy and the remainder, who fail to achieve a satisfactory response on this dose, require higher doses of up to 20 mg/kg daily for short periods. However, diphosphonate treatment may be combined with calcitonin to keep the dose below 5 mg/kg daily to prevent hypomineralisation from taking place. Side-effects include abdominal discomfort and diarrhoea.

7 The Endocrine Pancreas

The endocrine pancreas consists of the islets of Langerhans, the cells of which originate from the neuroectoderm and are part of the diffuse endocrine system (APUD cells). The islet is composed of four main types of cells: α-cells mainly secrete glucagon, β-cells secrete insulin, δ-cells secrete somatostatin and PP-cells pancreatic polypeptide. Whilst the physiological roles for glucagon and insulin are well recognised, the functions of the other two hormones are not clear.

Insulin is secreted as proinsulin which is cleaved to release equimolar amounts of insulin with the connecting peptide (C-peptide). Glucose is the main stimulus of insulin secretion which is direct into the portal vein. The liver extracts insulin at a variable rate depending on the nutritional state. The ratio of portal to peripheral insulin varies from 3 to 10:1 and this has important therapeutic implications when insulin is given directly into the peripheral circulation. Peripheral insulin is degraded by the liver and has a half-life of 5 minutes although its biological effects may last longer (up to 20 minutes). C-peptide is not metabolised by the liver so that its measurement in the peripheral circulation is a better estimate of β-cell function than peripheral insulin. C-peptide is metabolised by the kidney and has a half-life in the circulation of 20–35 minutes. There are three main target organs for insulin (Fig. 7.1):

1. The liver regulates glucose supplies to the tissues. In the *fed state* insulin levels rise, inhibiting hepatic glucose production from glycogenolysis and gluconeogenesis, and the liver converts incoming glucose to glycogen. Glycogen storage is limited and excess glucose is diverted into lipid synthesis. Lipid is secreted by the liver as very light density protein and transported to extra-hepatic sites for storage. In the *fasting state*, insulin secretion falls and hepatic glucose production increases.

2. In muscle, insulin promotes glucose transfer into cells, stimulating glycogen synthesis; inhibits fatty acid transport; increases amino acid transport and protein synthesis; and stimulates the entry of potassium into cells. In the fasting state, muscle derives 80% of its energy from fatty acids but in the fed state the energy supply is changed to glucose.

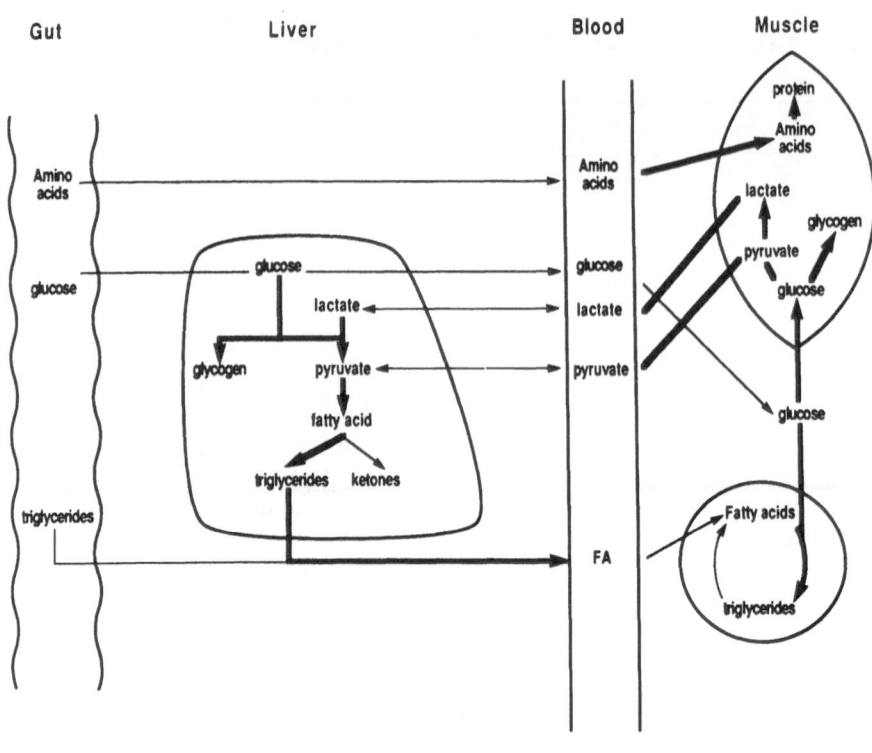

FED STATE   7.1a

Fig. 7.1. a The action of insulin on its three major targets: liver, muscle and fat (thick lines indicate stimulation and thinner lines indicate inhibition by insulin). **b** The action of counterregulatory hormones is to oppose the action of insulin to maintain blood glucose concentrations and protect the brain against hypoglycaemia. A, adrenaline; C, cortisol, G, glucagon. (Adapted from Baird JD and Alberti KGMM (1986). In: Edwards CRW (ed) Integrated clinical science: endocrinology. Heinemann, London, pp 133–197.)

3. In fat, lipolysis is inhibited at normal basal insulin levels; it is decreased even further in the fed state.

Whilst low levels of insulin inhibit lipolysis and hepatic glucose production, a two- to threefold increase in insulin secretion is required to increase glucose utilisation, protein synthesis and lipid synthesis to effect potassium transport. The action of insulin is antagonised by the catabolic hormones, glucagon, catecholamines, glucocorticoids and growth hormone. In the fasting state insulin levels fall and the effect of these hormones predominates, whereas in the fed state the effect of insulin predominates.

Glucose is derived from three sources: absorption from the gut, gly-cogenolysis (breakdown of glycogen) and gluconeogenesis (glucose produc-

Gut   Liver   Blood   Muscle

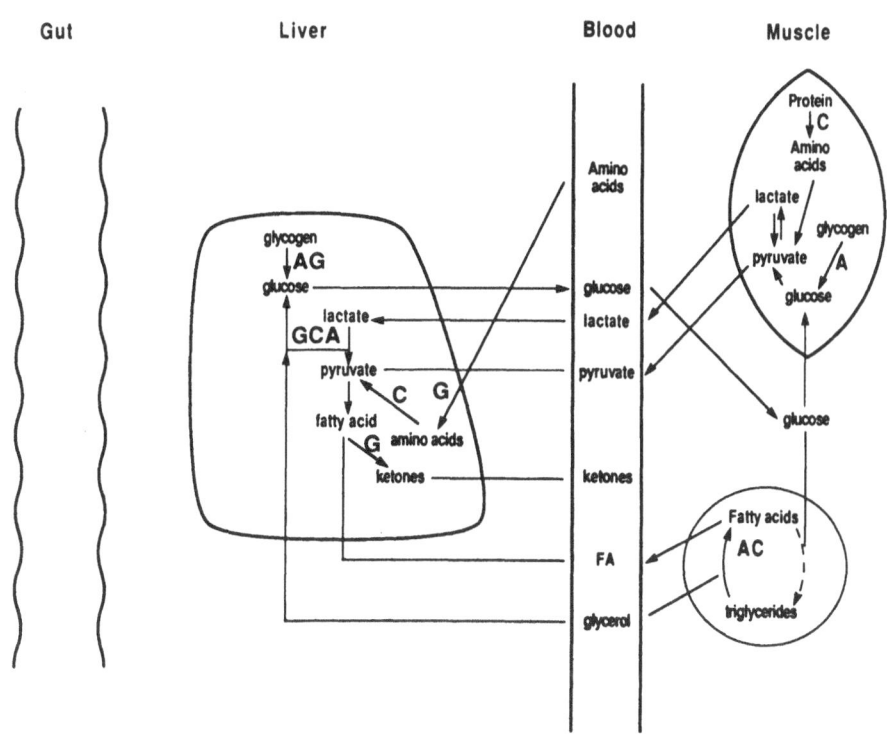

7.1b

tion from amino acids). Although most tissues have the enzyme required to synthesise and hydrolyse glycogen, only the liver and kidneys have the enzyme required to release glucose into the circulation (glucose-6-phosphatase). However, for practical purposes the liver is the sole source of endogenous glucose production.

Maintenance of normal blood glucose concentrations requires precise matching of glucose disposal to a combination of endogenous production and dietary sources. In the postabsorptive state (fasting or basal), hepatic glucose production and glucose disposal rates are equal and average 2.2 mg/kg/min. Of this, approximately 60% of glucose disposal is accounted for by the brain and the remainder is used by glycosylating tissues such as blood and kidney. About 75% of hepatic glucose production results from glycogenolysis and the remainder from gluconeogenesis of lactate, pyruvate, amino acids and glycerol representing 13%, 1%, 7% and 4% respectively of hepatic glucose production. Hepatic glycogen stores are approximately 70 g but soon fall to below 10 g after a prolonged fast (24 hours or more) so that gluconeogenesis becomes the major source of glucose. Thus muscle and protein are degraded and lipolysis accelerates to maintain blood glucose levels and ketones become a major source of fuel for the brain. In the fed state glucose absorption results in rates of exogenous glucose delivery that are double that of postabsorptive hepatic glucose production. As glucose is absorbed, increased insulin secretion inhibits hepatic glucose production and glucose disposal by liver, fat and muscle increases to maintain blood glucose concentrations at the postabsorptive level and to assimilate exogenous glucose. The maintenance of adequate blood glucose levels is the major purpose of glucose homeostasis since it is the main metabolic fuel of the brain and nervous tissue.

Glucose counterregulation is not due solely to the dissipation of insulin. Glucagon is the major counterregulatory hormone acutely stimulating glycogenolysis and chronically stimulating gluconeogenesis to increase hepatic glucose output. Adrenaline acts in concert with glucagon and may prevent hypoglycaemia when the action of glucagon alone may be insufficient. Thus hypoglycaemia can only occur in the presence of functionally adequate liver stores of glucose if either glucagon or adrenaline are insufficient and insulin is present, or there is excessive insulin action.

Hyperglycaemia

Diabetes mellitus is a syndrome characterised by reduced insulin action resulting in hyperglycaemia. It covers a heterogeneous group of disorders with widely varying aetiologies but these may be divided into three broad categories:

1. *Type I diabetes* has a prevalence of approximately 2 per 1000 and may present at any age with peaks in early childhood and adolescence. Destruction of β-cells results in insulin deficiency, and ketoacidosis will develop if the patient is not treated with insulin (insulin-dependent). It is usual to subdivide this category into an autoimmune group associated with a female preponderance, age at presentation over 35 years, permanent development of islet-cell antibodies, HLA type DR3 and often with other clinical autoimmune disorders, and a **non-autoimmune group** associated with equal sex incidence, age at presentation under 25 years, transient development of islet-cell antibodies, HLA type DR4 and development of insulin-binding antibodies following insulin treatment.

2. *Type II diabetes* is more common, with a prevalence of approximately 1% and a strong familial aggregation. The defect in islet-cell function is ill-understood: insulin secretion is reduced but sufficient to prevent ketoacidosis (non-insulin dependent) although some type II diabetics may require insulin to control hyperglycaemia (insulin-treated). Whilst it is usual to divide this group into obese (25%) and non-obese (75%) patients, all type II diabetics

show a degree of insulin resistance which is greater in obese than non-obese patients. In particular hepatic resistance to insulin in type II diabetes results in increased hepatic glucose production.

3. *Other causes* include pancreatic disease, endocrine conditions (cortico-steroid excess, phaeochromocytoma, acromegaly, glucagonoma and hyperthyroidism) and genetic disorders (DIDMOAD syndrome). Rare abnormalities of insulin receptors exist.

Diagnosis

The diagnosis must always be established by measuring the blood glucose level. A random whole blood glucose concentration in excess of 11 mmol/l is diagnostic of diabetes but for lower levels whole blood glucose concentrations should be obtained at 0 and 2 hours following the oral administration of 75 g glucose. It is important that patients should have eaten their normal diet prior to the test, which should be performed in the morning after an overnight fast. Respective fasting and 2-hour postglucose whole blood glucose levels of: <7 mmol/l are normal; <7 and >7–10 mmol/l respectively indicate impaired glucose tolerance; >7 and >10 mmol/l respectively indicate diabetes mellitus. (One mmol/l should be added to these figures if venous plasma is used.)

Treatment

Acute Hyperglycaemia

Acute hyperglycaemia may present as an emergency as diabetic ketoacidosis or hyperosmolar coma. There is probably no fundamental difference between these two states: in the former there is insufficient insulin to suppress hyperglycaemia and lipolysis whereas in the latter insulin deficiency is less marked. The low level of insulin is sufficient to prevent lipolysis but the deficiency severe enough to cause hyperglycaemia (Fig. 7.2). Ketoacidosis therefore occurs in the younger type I patient whilst hyperosmolar coma occurs in the elderly type II. The mortality from ketoacidosis remains as high as 5%–10% in specialist centres and may be as high as 25% elsewhere. The mortality from hyperosmolar coma is higher (40%–60%), reflecting the older age of the patient. The condition requires intensive medical and nursing care.

General measures should include nursing the patient in the semi-prone position if unconscious, until a nasogastric tube has been passed to aspirate the gastric contents. Infection is not usually a precipitating cause of diabetic ketoacidosis so that routine antibiotics are not indicated. Nevertheless a careful search should be made for evidence of infection, and if found appropriately treated. Confirmation of diabetic ketoacidosis can be made at the bedside estimating blood glucose levels with BM-glycaemie (Boehringer) 20–800 reagent strips using a reflectance meter and estimating blood ketones

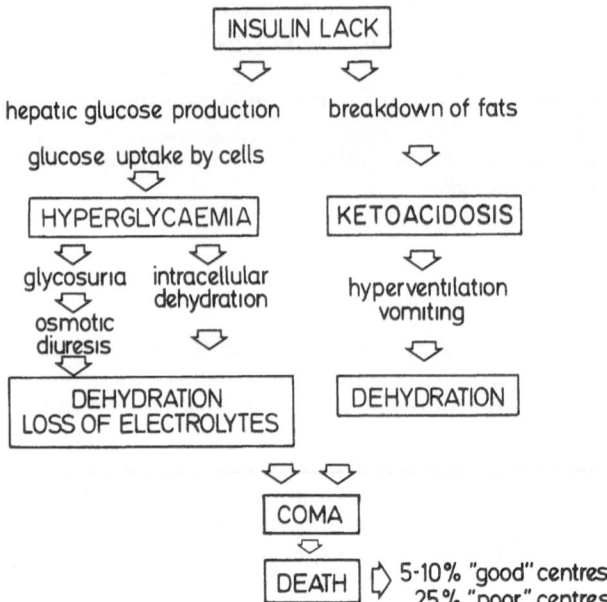

Fig. 7.2. The pathogenesis of diabetic ketoacidosis–hyperosmolar coma.

using plasma and Acetest tablets. Blood samples should be sent to the laboratory for more accurate assessment of blood glucose, electrolytes and arterial blood gases. Frequent and rapid biochemical testing is mandatory. Hypoxia should be treated with appropriate oxygen therapy. Anticoagulation with heparin should be considered in hyperosmolar coma because of an increased risk of thrombotic events. Disseminated intravascular coagulation is occasionally seen in diabetic ketoacidosis.

Specific measures are aimed at correction of fluid and electrolyte deficits, reduction of blood glucose concentrations and correction of acidosis.

1. *Fluid and electrolyte replacement* is assessed by clinical examination, pulse, supine and erect blood pressure, urine output and estimation of plasma electrolytes. It may be necessary to insert an indwelling urinary catheter if no urine is passed within 4 hours and, in patients where fluid replacement may present problems, monitoring of central venous pressure is needed. Due to the osmotic diuresis, vomiting and hyperventilation, patients with diabetic ketoacidosis are depleted of approximately 5–10 l of fluid (50% intra– and 50% extracellular fluid), 500 mmol sodium, 350 mmol chloride and 300–1000 mmol potassium. Urinary loss of potassium is accounted for by insulin deficiency, acidosis and secondary hyperaldosteronism. A regimen for

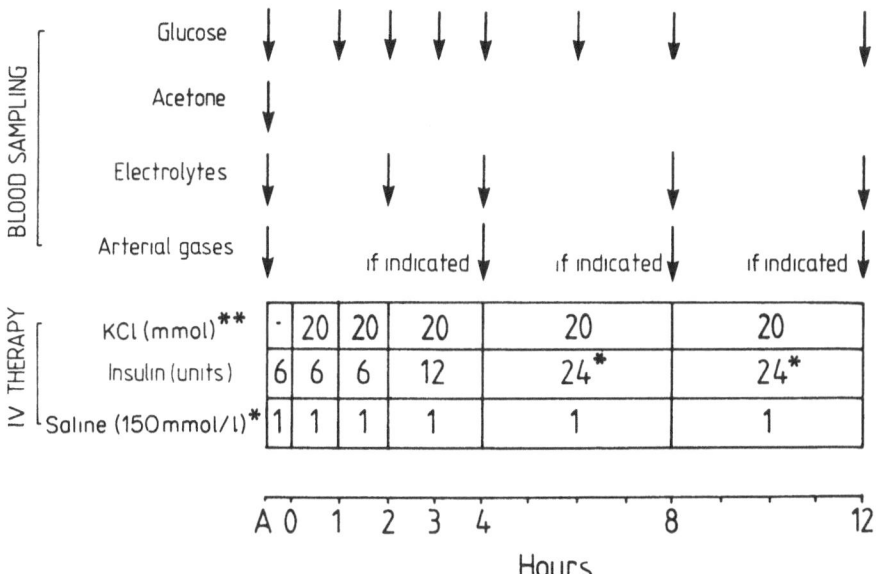

Fig. 7.3. A regimen for the treatment of diabetic ketoacidosis (* if plasma sodium exceeds 150 mmol/l, the fluid should be changed to either half-physiological saline if the blood glucose is >10 mmol/l or 10% glucose if the blood glucose is <10 mmol/l; ** the amount of potassium may need to be adjusted according to the plasma potassium concentrations).

intravenous fluid and electrolyte replacement is illustrated in Fig. 7.3. Despite a greater loss of water than of sodium, physiological saline (150 mmol/l) is the correct replacement fluid to prevent dangerous fluid shifts. However, if plasma sodium concentrations exceed 150 mmol/l, half-physiological saline (75 mmol/l) is indicated if the blood glucose is in excess of 10 mmol/l; 10% glucose (with insulin) may be given if the blood glucose level is below this. In hyperosmolar coma over 50% of patients will have a normal or elevated plasma sodium concentration, so that replacement with half-physiological saline is often necessary. The rate of fluid administration is such as to correct severe dehydration as rapidly as possible; 1 litre is given in the first 30 minutes whilst awaiting the results of biochemistry, 2 litres in the next 2 hours and 1 litre in the succeeding 2 hours. This regimen may be modified according to the severity of dehydration.

Although most patients have a normal or high plasma potassium concentration on admission, potassium administration is needed early in therapy to correct the serious potassium loss and to prevent hypokalaemia occurring as a result of rehydration and insulin administration. Potassium may be given as soon as the plasma potassium is known and therapy monitored on the basis of biochemistry. Usually 20 mmol is given hourly in the first 4 hours but the rate may be increased to 40 mmol hourly if the plasma potassium is below 3 mmol/l, or reduced to 10 mmol hourly for levels of 5-6 mmol/l. Up to 70% of intravenous potassium is lost by urinary excretion in the first 24 hours and it is fruitless to attempt total replacement during this time. After acute therapy, oral potassium should be given for 10 days.

2. *Correction of hyperglycaemia and acidosis* is achieved by the continuous intravenous administration of low-dose highly purified short-acting insulin. In the average patient with ketoacidosis plasma insulin levels are approximately 10 mU/l (similar to normal fasting levels), indicating a relative rather than absolute deficiency of insulin imposed by circulating stress hormones. Insulin should be given in a dose to achieve plasma concentrations in excess of 50 mU/l. Each unit of insulin administered per hour will achieve a plasma concentration of 20 mU/l so that a rate of 6 units per hour is more than sufficient to suppress lipolysis. As with all forms of continuous intravenous therapy, care must be taken to ensure there is no interruption in delivery. This can be achieved by adding the insulin to the intravenous fluids. Adsorption of insulin to plastic and glass is a potential problem but is clinically rarely important. This regimen should lower the blood glucose level by approximately 5 mmol/l per hour in a predictable manner. Once a blood glucose concentration of 10 mmol/l has been attained the intravenous fluid should be changed from saline to 10% glucose and the insulin infusion rate reduced to 3 units per hour and adjusted to maintain a blood glucose of 6-8 mmol/l. The insulin/glucose/potassium infusion should be continued until the acidosis is clinically and biochemically corrected and the patient ready to take normal meals with subcutaneous insulin.

The intravenous administration of bicarbonate is rarely if ever indicated. Potential dangers of bicarbonate administration include a paradoxical rise in CNS hydrogen ion concentration, sodium overload, hypokalaemia and tissue hypoxia secondary to impaired oxygenated haemoglobin dissociation. If the patient is shocked and severely acidotic with arterial hydrogen ion levels in excess of 100 mmol/l, 500 ml of 2.6% sodium bicarbonate may be given intravenously. However it is debatable whether the administration of bicarbonate will have any beneficial effect on the clinical outcome.

Chronic Hyperglycaemia

Chronic hyperglycaemia is only one facet of diabetes mellitus. However, glucose is one of the few metabolites that is easily measured and current aims in treatment are to establish as near normoglycaemia as possible and to prevent long-term complications. These include macroangiopathy (atherosclerosis), microangiopathy (retinopathy and nephropathy) and neuropathy; the development of microvascular complications and neuropathy appears to be related to the duration of diabetes and the quality of blood glucose control.

Type I diabetes is treated by combination of diet and insulin. The role of **dietary measures** is important in the control of insulin-dependent diabetes. Current recommendations are based on the quantity, quality and distribution of the diet. The quantity (energy content) of the diet should be related to the individual and should allow maintenance of an appropriate body weight and a lifestyle of his or her choosing. The quality of the diet should be that recommended for a non-diabetic but with a few minor restrictions; its basis is a lowered fat, increased carbohydrate, high fibre diet.

The total carbohydrate content of the diet should provide approximately 50% of the total energy. Carbohydrate should be in the form of slowly absorbed polysaccharides, and foods containing simple sugars (mono- and disaccharides in sweets, chocolates and sweetened drinks) should be excluded as they are rapidly absorbed and cause wide fluctuations in glucose control. Foods rich in fibre (wholemeal bread, wholewheat pasta, wholegrain or fibre-enriched cereals, brown rice, vegetables, beans, fruit and fibre-rich biscuits) are to be encouraged as there is clear evidence that suitable dietary fibre in meals delays glucose absorption and may prevent hypoglycaemia in insulin-treated patients. It is better to choose high-fibre foods than to add extra fibre to the diet by means that are often expensive, cumbersome or unpalatable. Special diabetic foods containing sorbitol and fructose as glucose substitutes are of little health benefit. Saccharin is an acceptable sugar substitute. Ordinary alcoholic drinks may be consumed by diabetics provided the energy contribution is taken into account. A reduction in fat intake is important because of its long-term benefit with regard to macroangiopathy. If possible the total fat intake should represent 35% of the total energy requirement; polyunsaturated fats are preferable to saturated animal fats. However, there is little justification in imposing such rigid requirements on elderly established diabetics as the benefits are long term rather than short term.

It is essential that diabetics receiving insulin should be advised on the distribution of their diet and the timing of general food choices or carbohydrate exchanges. The need for a regular pattern of feeding should be stressed in order to prevent hypoglycaemia, but appropriate advice can be given on adjusting the timing of insulin injection to match social needs of altered meal times or shift work. It is traditional to advise that most of the carbohydrate be taken at the three main meals—breakfast, lunch and dinner—but these are not necessarily times when according to blood sugar profiles most carbohydrate is needed. Less carbohydrate at breakfast and more at mid-morning improves blood sugar control. Great effort should be made to tailor the diet to the patient's own lifestyle, but snacks between meals at mid-morning, mid-afternoon and bedtime are particularly important in preventing hypoglycaemia.

Insulins may be classified according to their source, purity and duration of action:

1. *Source.* Until recently all insulin used was extracted from the pancreas of either cow or pig. Bovine insulin differs from human insulin in two amino acid sequences of the A-chain, whereas porcine insulin differs from human insulin in only one amino acid on the B-chain. Bovine insulin is therefore potentially more antigenic than porcine insulin. Human insulin has recently been prepared by two different methods. The first is enzymatic manipulation of the

differing amino acid on the B-chain of porcine insulin (semi-synthetic); the second uses recombinant DNA technology to instruct *E. coli* to produce human insulin. The potency of the insulins prepared by these two methods is similar and there is no significant difference in biological activity in humans.

2. *Purity*. Insulins differ in their purity and it is probably the presence of contaminants rather than the species of insulin that is responsible for antigenicity and the development of anti-insulin antibodies in insulin-treated patients. Conventional bovine and porcine insulins contain significant contaminants such as proinsulin (40 000 ppm), insulin fragments and other pancreatic hormones. But in purified bovine and porcine insulins obtained by gel filtration chromatography proinsulin contamination is reduced to less than 50 ppm; and highly purified insulins have been obtained by ion exchange chromatography which reduces proinsulin contamination to below 10 ppm. Human insulins are highly purified by their method of manufacture. It is debatable whether insulin antibodies are of clinical significance. There is no evidence to suggest that the development of anti-insulin antibodies is responsible for long-term diabetic complications. However, highly purified (human) insulins are less likely to cause allergic reactions and fat atrophy at the site of injection. It would seem wise to use these highly purified human preparations for all new patients, for those requiring intermittent insulin therapy (pregnancy and surgery), and for established insulin-treated diabetics who require better control or suffer from fat atrophy.

3. *Duration of action*. The other property to be considered in the choice of insulin is the speed and duration of action, as well as the route of administration. A short-acting insulin, such as Actrapid (Novo), has a plasma half-life of 5 minutes with a biological half-life of approximately 20 minutes when given intravenously. Therefore it must be given continuously if this route is used to produce a sustained effect. When given intramuscularly the half-life is prolonged to 2 hours but absorption may be impaired in circulatory collapse. The subcutaneous route is employed for maintenance therapy; the time to onset of action is approximately 30 minutes with a duration of 6 hours. Factors influencing absorption of insulin from subcutaneous sites include depth of injection, massage, exercise, local degradation and site (absorption from abdomen>arm>thigh). It is very important that the patient employs a consistent attitude to injection technique in order to achieve consistent blood sugar control. Insulin may be modified to prolong its time to onset and duration of action by the preparation of insulin–zinc suspensions. A medium-acting insulin, such as Monotard (Novo), has a time to onset of action of 1–3 hours with a duration of action of 7–15 hours, and a long-acting insulin, such as Ultratard (Novo), has a time to onset of 3 hours with a duration of 10–24 hours.

Most insulin-dependent diabetics who wish to achieve a good **blood glucose control regimen** require twice-daily injections of a combination of short- and medium-acting insulins, taken 30 minutes before breakfast and the evening meal (Fig. 7.4D). These insulins may be mixed in one syringe provided they

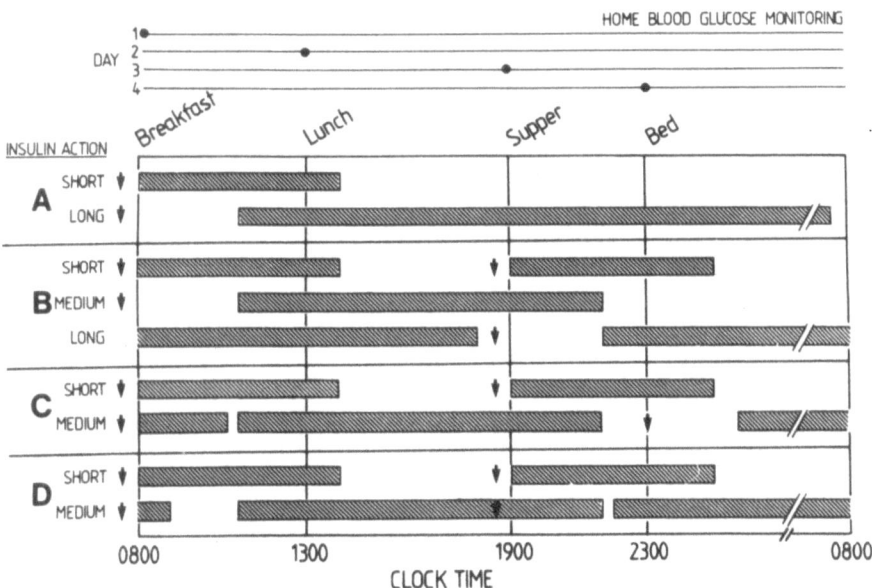

Fig. 7.4. Examples of four insulin regimens: A, the administration of a short- and a long-acting insulin once daily is particularly suitable for elderly diabetics in whom strict glucose is not needed; B, the administration of a short- and medium-acting insulin in the morning with a short- and long-acting insulin in the evening is one way to overcome the dawn phenomenon; C, the administration of a short- and medium-acting insulin in the morning with a short-acting insulin in the evening and a medium-acting insulin as a third injection on retiring is another way of overcoming the dawn phenomenon; D, conventional administration on a short- and medium-acting insulin twice daily is suitable for the majority of insulin-treated diabetics.

are injected immediately; otherwise the zinc suspension may affect the action of the short-acting insulin.

One problem encountered with this regimen is hyperglycaemia before breakfast, which cannot be controlled by appropriate increases in the dose of the evening medium-acting insulin as this results in nocturnal hypoglycaemia. The evening medium-acting insulin is insufficient to cover the early-morning rise in insulin requirements caused by increased secretion of insulin antagonists, particularly GH (dawn phenomenon). This can be overcome either by substituting a long-acting insulin for the medium-acting evening insulin (Fig. 7.4B) or by rescheduling the evening medium-acting insulin to be given as a third injection last thing at night before retiring (Fig. 7.4C). In older patients, where less rigorous control is needed, once-daily injection with a long-acting insulin is often sufficient (Fig. 7.4A).

The dose of insulin should be adjusted according to the blood sugar control. This can be assessed by home blood glucose monitoring employing BM-Test-Glycaemie 20-800 (Boehringer) reagent strips with or without a reflectance meter. Estimation of blood glucose concentrations by this method is simple and reliable and is largely replacing urinary glucose methods, which are inaccurate in reflecting blood glucose levels. Blood is obtained by a finger prick before each of the four meal times but testing can be restricted to one test per day by staggering it in a systematic way. Insulin dosages should be adjusted gradually in order to correct trends in blood glucose levels, the aim being to maintain values between 4 and 6 mmol/l. It is sensible to adjust only one dose each time.

Long-term blood glucose control can be assessed by estimation of glycosylated haemoglobin A_1 concentrations. Irreversible glycosylation of haemoglobin occurs during synthesis of the protein and the degree of glycosylation is dependent on the blood glucose concentration prevailing at the time. The percentage of haemoglobin A_1 glycosylated (normal range 6%–8%) gives an integrated picture of the average blood glucose levels during the life span of a red cell (120 days). Unlike blood glucose estimations this value does not fluctuate from day to day, but care must be taken in interpreting these results in the presence of haemolysis, haemoglobinopathies or renal failure. The aim of insulin therapy is to normalise blood glucose concentrations, haemoglobin A_1 and blood lipids whilst keeping the patient free from hypoglycaemia.

In recent years a great deal of research has been devoted to the development of new insulin delivery systems. **Continuous subcutaneous insulin infusion** employs a small portable infusion pump that delivers short-acting insulin at a basal rate (15 mU/kg/h) with facilities for a preprandial boost. A fine-gauge needle is inserted under the skin and is changed daily. Whilst this system can normalise metabolic profiles when compared with conventional multiple injections it is not known whether this confers any advantage in the long term. Hypoglycaemia and ketoacidosis occur less frequently in pump-treated patients than conventionally treated ones, but pump failure can be a problem. Complexity and cost prohibit routine use of the system.

An **alternative route for insulin delivery** is via the peritoneal cavity, to produce a more physiological ratio of portal to peripheral insulin. Current evidence suggests that raised peripheral insulin levels, an inevitable consequence of conventional insulin treatment, increase the synthesis and deposition of lipid in arterial walls, contributing to the long-term complication of macroangiopathy.

Pancreatic transplantation is still beset with formidable problems.

Insulin-induced hypoglycaemia is a major hazard of conventional insulin treatment and all diabetics treated with insulin should be taught about the causes, symptoms and treatment. Relatives and friends should also be trained in its treatment. The patient should always carry Dextrosol tablets or Lucozade to abort any hypoglycaemic episode before it becomes serious. Relatives can help an unconscious patient by maintaining a patent airway, calling immediate medical help and by giving glucagon 1 mg by intramuscular injection, provided of course that the patient has been issued with it. Hypoglycaemia causing unconsciousness should be confirmed at the bedside with BM-Test-Glycaemie 20-800 reagent strips and immediately treated with

20–50 ml 50% glucose administered intravenously. Cerebral oedema resulting from prolonged hypoglycaemia can be treated with dexamethasone 4 mg 6-hourly by intramuscular injection. Because of the risk of hypoglycaemia, diabetics in Britain must notify both their insurance company and the Driver and Vehicle Licensing Centre, Swansea, SA99 1AR, if they drive. The possibility of hypoglycaemia should also be considered in relation to employment or hobbies—whether resulting mental confusion might threaten the safety of the patient or others has to be considered.

It is wise to **store stocks of insulin** in the refrigerator, but insulin solutions contain a preservative and are stable at room temperature in the British climate for several months. Insulin is currently prescribed in a strength of 100 U/ml and glass syringes are available marked directly in units for 100 U/ml insulin. Disposable plastic syringes have the advantage of being re-usable for up to a week if kept in the fridge, and are freely available under the NHS.

Type II diabetes is treated by dietary measures with or without an oral hypoglycaemic drug (30% of cases) but occasionally treatment with insulin is necessary to control hyperglycaemia even though such patients are not necessarily insulin-dependent.

Obese diabetics are treated with weight reduction as the main goal. There should be a reduction in the energy content of the diet with special emphasis on fat reduction, a proportionally more generous allowance of carbohydrate and the elimination of simple sugars. Patients should be seen at monthly intervals by the dietitian to encourage weight loss. An average patient will lose approximately 2 kg per week with greater weight loss at the beginning than at the end. It is often difficult for the patient to achieve ideal body weight and some compromise can be reached if the degree of blood glucose control is satisfactory. If there is a failure to achieve reasonable weight loss the addition of the oral hypoglycaemic agent metformin to the treatment regimen should be considered. Metformin is a biguanide inhibiting hepatic glucose production with a resulting fall in blood glucose levels. It has several unpleasant side-effects including anorexia, malaise, vomiting and diarrhoea and it is probably these properties that permit weight loss despite improved blood glucose control. Lactic acidosis is a potential and more serious side-effect and metformin should not be prescribed in patients with either liver disease or renal impairment (the drug is excreted in the urine unchanged). Doses should not exceed 850 mg 12-hourly. If blood glucose levels still remain high, the only options left are combined treatment with a sulphonylurea or insulin treatment. Unfortunately either of these measures will result in significant weight gain to compound the problem, so that maximal effort should be made to control the obese patient with diet, with or without metformin.

Non-obese diabetics are treated with a diet of sufficient energy content to maintain an ideal body weight but additional treatment with a sulphonylurea is necessary if the patient is significantly underweight or blood glucose control is poor. Sulphonylureas act in two ways: they increase insulin secretion in response to glucose and enhance insulin action. Selecting a sulphonylurea is largely a matter of personal choice. Rare side-effects include rashes, jaundice and agranulocytosis. Aspirin, sulphonamides and monoamine oxidase inhibitors may potentiate the action of sulphonylureas. Chlorpropamide has a long duration of action with a biological half-life of 36 hours and may cause hypoglycaemia, particularly at night, flushing with alcohol and enhancement of the renal response to vasopressin causing a dilutional hyponatraemia. It is excreted in the urine and should not be prescribed in renal failure. It is administered in doses of 100–375 mg once daily. Glipizide is an alternative drug with a much shorter half-life of approximately 5 hours and is more suitable for elderly patients. It is given in doses of 2.5–10 mg 8-hourly by mouth. If blood glucose control is unsatisfactory on a sulphonylurea alone, combination with metformin may be helpful but often this is an indication for insulin treatment. Approximately 30% of patients treated with sulphonylureas will require insulin within 5 years. Adequate control is assessed by home estimations of fasting blood glucose, and levels of haemoglobin A_1 and blood lipids.

Long-term Complications

The long-term complications of diabetes are best treated by prevention, but it is not yet known whether current efforts to tighten blood glucose control will achieve this end. Type I diabetes is associated with an increased mortality of five times that of the general population with death under the age of 50 attributable to macroangiopathy (myocardial infarction 35% and strokes 7% of deaths), microangiopathy (renal failure 17% of deaths) and metabolic comas (20%).

The average life expectancy of a type I diabetic is 30 years from diagnosis and only 50% will reach 50 years of age. In terms of morbidity nearly 30% will be registered blind, 30% will develop renal failure due to microangiopathy and 10% will require an amputation for a combination of neuropathy and macroangiopathy. The mortality from type II diabetes is probably 1.5 times that of the general population and these patients can develop all the complications seen in their type I counterparts.

Diabetic eye disease should be monitored by routine assessment of visual acuity and the eye then dilated with a short-acting agent, tropicamide, prior to ophthalmoscopy.

1. *Lens opacities* are treated by cataract extraction.

2. *Simple retinopathy*, consisting of microaneurysms, haemorrhages and both "hard" and "soft" exudates, is often present without interference with vision and requires no treatment. "Soft" exudates indicate retinal ischaemia and are more worrying; they may herald the development of proliferative retinopathy. The development of maculopathy with encroachment of "hard" exudates or oedema onto the macula is an indication for photocoagulation. No benefit from this treatment is seen if the acuity has deteriorated to more than 6/36.

3. *Proliferative retinopathy* is characterised by neovascularisation with or without preretinal haemorrhages. Photocoagulation is of significant benefit in

treating proliferative retinopathy, particularly in those patients with new vessels on the disc and those who have sustained a vitreous haemorrhage. Untreated, 30% will be blind in 3 years. Photocoagulation can be achieved using either a xenon or an argon laser. The xenon beam is absorbed by the pigment layer of the retina and results in a full thickness burn of the retina; areas of coagulation are replaced by retinal glial tissue. This source is therefore useful for peripheral ablation of the retina to destroy any friable new vessels that may bleed into the vitreous space and to destroy areas of ischaemia that are a potential source of these new vessels. The argon beam is absorbed by haemoglobin and is therefore more accurate and may be better used for vessels near the optic disc. The treatment reduces a 3-year loss of acuity from 6/9 to 6/36, to 6/12. Vitreous haemorrhages can be treated surgically.

Nephropathy is an insidious disorder commencing with hypertrophy of glomeruli, increased glomerular filtration and microalbuminuria. These early defects can be reversed by meticulous blood glucose control. Proteinuria increases to become detectable by Albustix and does not often exceed 5 g per day. Renal function is often maintained for several years. When plasma creatinine concentrations exceed 200 μmol/l, the rate of increase can be used to predict the rate of progression of the disease. The patient usually becomes symptomatic once these concentrations exceed 500 μmol/l, with pulmonary oedema, peripheral oedema and anaemia. Declining renal function is complicated by hypertension. Hyporeninaemic hypoaldosteronism is common in diabetic nephropathy and usually results from damage to the juxtaglomerular apparatus. Hyperkalaemia and a hyperchloraemic acidosis are clues to the diagnosis. Once the stage of renal failure is reached the majority of patients suffer from other features of microangiopathy (80% have proliferative retinopathy), neuropathy, and many have features of macroangiopathy with ischaemic heart disease and amputations. The treatment of choice for end-stage renal failure is renal transplantation, with a graft survival rate of 33% and a patient survival rate of 42% at 2 years. If high-dose steroids are used to combat rejection, it is wise to anticipate increasing insulin requirements of approximately 20%. Alternative treatment is with haemodialysis or chronic ambulatory peritoneal dialysis. Insulin may be given in the peritoneal dialysis fluid providing absorption across the peritoneal membrane is satisfactory.

Neuropathy is either diffuse, affecting peripheral nerves and the autonomic nervous system, or localised, affecting single nerves and nerve roots.

1. *Diffuse peripheral neuropathy* is usually asymptomatic, mostly sensory, and affects the legs. With progression the patient may notice sensory loss and eventually 25% of diabetics of 20 years duration and over the age of 40 develop traumatic ulceration of the feet. Repeated trauma to the sole of the foot, usually under the first metatarsal head, causes painless ulceration and predisposes to infection and osteomyelitis. Abnormal mechanical stresses, normally prevented by pain, may damage joints in the foot (Charcot's joints). Joints most commonly affected are tarsometatarsal, metatarsophalangeal and

ankle. Patients at risk must be instructed in foot hygiene and advised on well-fitting shoes. A chiropodist should be an integral part of the diabetic clinic. Foot ulcers should be assessed in conjunction with a surgeon. Radiology of the foot is essential to determine whether there is underlying osteomyelitis, and wound swabs should be taken for bacteriology. Simple ulcers are best treated with bed rest. The wound can be kept clean with twice-daily irrigations of 2% Milton solution. Subsequently a walking plaster or crutches will allow the patient some mobility whilst keeping pressure off the ulcer. Specially made shoes are essential once the patient is more mobile. Any evidence of infection should be treated with appropriate antibiotics. Surgery is indicated for extensive infection or osteomyelitis. Every attempt should be made to achieve good blood glucose control in these patients. Seven per cent of patients develop a painful neuropathy, a miserable condition characterised by hypersensitivity to touch, paraesthesiae, pain and weight loss. Treatment of the condition is extremely difficult. Diabetic control should be as tight as possible, regular analgesia should be given and treatment with imipramine 75–150 mg daily is the treatment of choice. Phenothiazines or carbamazepine can also be helpful.

2. *Single nerve neuropathies* are often rapid in onset, severe and resolve within a year. Femoral neuropathy produces pain, muscle wasting and absent knee jerks (amyotrophy). Root pain may cause pain in the trunk, and cranial nerve lesions present as diplopia with third- or sixth-nerve palsies and often pain behind the eye. Complete recovery occurs spontaneously.

3. *Autonomic neuropathy* may result in postural hypotension, diarrhoea, delayed gastric emptying, impotence and urinary retention. Postural hypotension is uncommon and is treated with volume expansion with oral fludrocortisone up to 0.2 mg daily. Diabetic diarrhoea should be treated with codeine phosphate as required to control symptoms and three doses of tetracycline 250 mg, given at the onset, may halt an attack. Delayed gastric emptying can be improved by metoclopramide 10 mg 8-hourly by mouth. Urinary retention is treated with cholinergic drugs such as bethanecol 10–30 mg 8-hourly by mouth, but dilatation and resection of the bladder neck may have to be considered. Impotence may occur in up to 50% of diabetics with longstanding disease and results from psychological factors, macroangiopathy involving the internal pudendal artery and autonomic failure. Skilled and sympathetic counselling is required and any psychological element identified and treated if possible. Currently, impotence in diabetics is not curable although it is possible to supply a surgical implant to provide adequate vaginal penetration.

Special Problems of Diabetics

Some special problems encountered by diabetics include:

1. *Surgery.* The principle of glucose/insulin/potassium infusion can be applied to insulin-treated diabetics undergoing major surgery. For elective

operations the patient should be first on the list in the morning if possible. On the evening prior to operation, the normal dose of short-acting insulin is given with 50% of the medium-acting one. In the morning, blood is taken for estimation of blood glucose and electrolytes prior to the intravenous infusion of 500 ml 10% glucose containing 18 units short-acting insulin and 20 mmol potassium chloride over 6 hours. Blood glucose should be checked every 2 hours and appropriate changes in the insulin dose made. The infusion should never be stopped and other fluids may be given in addition if required but those containing lactate should be avoided because of the risk of lactic acidosis. After recovery the regimen can be continued until the patient is eating and the subcutaneous regimen recommenced. Patients undergoing minor operations can be treated by reducing the medium-acting insulin the night before and omitting the insulin on the morning of the operation. A short-acting insulin can then be given with food when the patient returns from theatre. The management of diabetics treated with diet or oral agents undergoing surgery is relatively simple providing the control is satisfactory prior to operation. Oral therapy should be discontinued on the day of operation and postoperative hyperglycaemia treated with subcutaneous insulin.

2. *Pregnancy* both complicates, and is complicated by, pre-existing diabetes. Maternal mortality, perinatal mortality and the number of congenital malformations are all increased when compared with a non-diabetic pregnancy. Maternal mortality results from metabolic deaths and infection. Established retinopathy and nephropathy may deteriorate during pregnancy and whilst retinopathy can be treated with photocoagulation, patients with nephropathy should be discouraged from becoming pregnant because of a threefold risk of pre-eclampsia and a shortened life in which to bring up the child. The pregnancy may be complicated by polyhydramnios, pre-eclampsia and an enlarged fetus. Fetal growth is stimulated by excessive fetal insulin, secreted in response to maternal hyperglycaemia. The cause of increased perinatal mortality is multifactorial, resulting from congenital malformations, sudden fetal death at 36–38 weeks and the respiratory distress syndrome. The cause of sudden intrauterine death is not known but probably relates to poor metabolic control. Neonatal respiratory distress occurs in premature infants deficient in pulmonary surfactant. Infants born to diabetic women have an increased risk of respiratory distress when compared with infants of the same gestational age born to normal women, and the problem is exacerbated by premature delivery, either elective to avoid sudden intrauterine death, or spontaneous.

There has been a fall in perinatal mortality over the past 50 years from 50% to approximately 4%. This is attributable to better diabetic control, permitting a more normal pregnancy which is allowed to go to term without increased risk of sudden fetal death and neonatal respiratory distress. Unfortunately, despite this decline, congenital malformations have appeared as the single most important cause of perinatal mortality, accounting for nearly half of the deaths. The cause of this is not known, nor whether the teratogenic factor operates before or after conception.

All pre-existing diabetics and patients developing diabetes in pregnancy (gestational diabetes) should be treated with insulin before and during a planned pregnancy. Diabetic control should be optimal for several months before conception with home blood glucose estimations between 4 and 6 mmol/l and a normal haemoglobin A_1 value. Good diabetic control can only be achieved with two or more insulin injections per day. From about 16 weeks onwards progressive insulin resistance develops requiring an increase in the dose of insulin. In addition, an increase in dietary requirements is needed to meet a normal weight gain of 12.5 kg during pregnancy. Blood glucose levels should be estimated four times a day and the patient reviewed monthly in a joint clinic with the obstetrician during the first two trimesters then weekly thereafter. Fetal gestation should be assessed and monitored with ultrasound, and fetal activity by regular assessment of fetal heart rate with particular attention to beat-to-beat variation. Preterm delivery at 38 weeks is indicated if there are problems but a well-controlled diabetic pregnancy can proceed to term. Vaginal delivery is preferred.

On the day of delivery normal insulin is discontinued and a 10% glucose/insulin/potassium infusion is employed at a rate of 500 ml 6-hourly with 6 units of short-acting insulin and 20 mmol of potassium chloride. Blood glucose levels are measured hourly by reflectance meter and insulin dose adjusted accordingly. Before and following delivery there is an immediate increase in insulin sensitivity and the dose of insulin infused will have to be reduced. It may take 24 hours before the insulin dose returns to its prepregnancy level. In cases of gestational diabetes, glucose tolerance may return to normal and should be assessed by a glucose tolerance test at 6 weeks.

3. *Contraceptive advice* to diabetics is similar to that for non-diabetics. Barrier methods may be preferred because of doubts over safety of the oral contraceptive pill. If the combined pill is desired, a small increase in the dose of insulin may be needed in insulin-treated diabetics. A progestogen-only pill is probably preferable, particularly in gestational diabetics. Intrauterine contraceptive devices are best avoided because of the risk of pelvic infection.

Hypoglycaemia

Hypoglycaemia is defined as a blood glucose concentration of less than 2.2 mmol/l and can be divided into two groups: fasting hypoglycaemia and postprandial hypoglycaemia.

Diagnosis

Postabsorptive (fasting) hypoglycaemia is the most common form and offending agents include insulin, sulphonylureas and alcohol. Endogenous hyperinsulinism is rare, occurring in one person per million, and is due to an insulin-secreting tumour of the pancreas (insulinoma) in approximately 75% of cases. Insulinomas present in both sexes with an average age of 50 years in sporadic cases but at a younger age (23 years) in those patients with a multiple endocrine syndrome (MEN 1: primary hyperparathyroidism, pituitary tumour and pancreatic islet cell tumour). Ninety-nine per cent of cases are confined to the pancreas; they are usually 1–2 cm in diameter and 10% are malignant. Hyperinsulinism also occurs in the absence of an insulinoma and is probably due to β-cell hyperplasia and occurs with antibodies to insulin or its receptor. Other causes of fasting hypoglycaemia include liver disease (including glycogen storage diseases, lack of counterregulatory hormones (particularly cortisol and growth hormone) and mesenchymal malignancies.

The first step in the management of a suspected patient is to establish the relationship of any symptoms to documented spontaneous hypoglycaemia. Obvious causes such as drugs and adrenocortical insufficiency should be excluded. At the time of a spontaneous hypoglycaemic episode, blood should be taken for plasma insulin and C-peptide estimations in order to determine the presence of endogenous hyperinsulinaemia. In these cases, plasma insulin levels are inappropriately high for the prevailing blood glucose level and concurrent estimation of C-peptide confirms the source of insulin as endogenous. If the patient fails to develop spontaneous hypoglycaemia whilst under investigation, an insulin hypoglycaemia test should be performed (see Chapter 5) with estimation of blood glucose and plasma C-peptide levels. Hypoglycaemia will suppress endogenous insulin secretion in normal individuals and therefore under these circumstances, and providing adequate hypoglycaemia has been achieved, a plasma C-peptide in excess of 1.5 ng/ml is indicative of endogenous hyperinsulinism. Further investigation should be aimed at localisation of the tumour with transhepatic venous sampling for plasma insulin levels (Fig. 7.5). Computerised tomography is of limited value because of the small size of these tumours. However, computerised tomography may be of use in searching for metastatic spread and further tests should be performed to exclude the possibility of a multiple endocrine syndrome.

Postprandial (reactive) hypoglycaemia occurs exclusively after meals and usually within a few hours of eating. Commonly this occurs following gastric surgery and in patients with errors of carbohydrate metabolism. Diagnosis is confirmed by an extended (3-hour) glucose tolerance test.

Treatment

Insulinomas are best treated by surgical removal where possible. Where surgery is not possible, treatment with diazoxide can be very effective but associated fluid retention may require treatment with a diuretic. Long-acting analogues of somatostatin may also prove to be of value by inhibiting insulin secretion.

Postprandial hypoglycaemia responds well to dietary measures consisting of exclusion of sucrose and frequent regular meals, high in fibre.

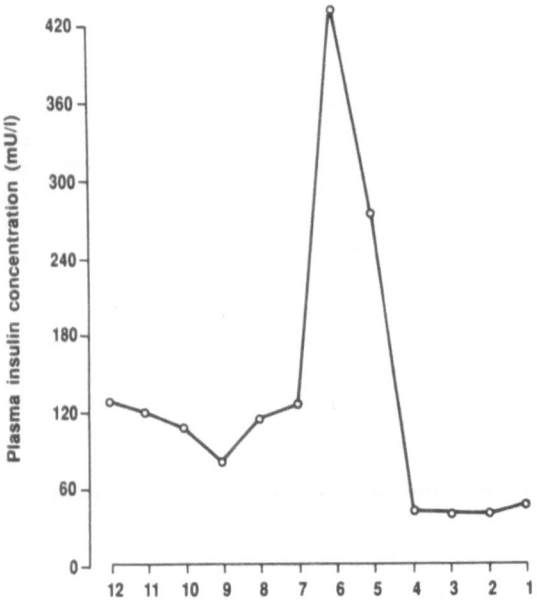

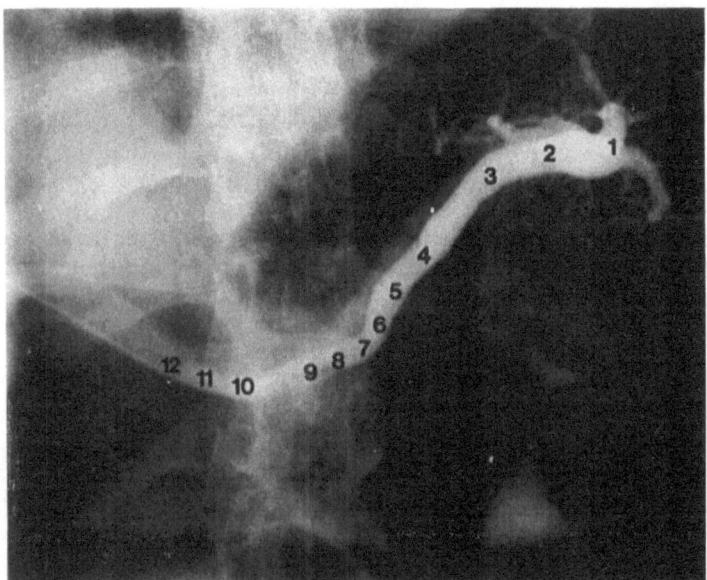

Fig. 7.5. Transhepatic portal venous sampling for plasma insulin levels in a patient with an insulinoma.

SECTION II
Clinical Pharmacology of Endocrine Drugs

8 Clinical Pharmacology

Allan D. Struthers

General Principles

An oral dose of any drug has to surmount a series of barriers before it can enter the systemic circulation and thereafter exert its therapeutic effect. The first problems are the dissolution of the drug in the gut lumen and the passage of the drug across the gut epithelium into the portal circulation. The latter part of this process is facilitated by the degree of lipophilicity of the drug. For a large number of endocrine treatments (insulin, calcitonin and vasopressin), the active ingredient cannot withstand the adverse environment of the gut lumen so that this very first step becomes an insurmountable obstacle.

The second main obstacle lies in the enzymes in the liver and gut wall which are capable of metabolising the incoming drug before it has even reached the arterial plasma. This is called presystemic metabolism and ironically those lipophilic drugs which are best absorbed by the gut wall are precisely those drugs which are subject to the greatest presystemic metabolism. Bromocriptine is one endocrine drug which is subject to enormous first-pass metabolism, with 94% of the absorbed dose being so metabolised.

Therefore between gut lumen and arterial plasma there are huge barriers. The bioavailability of a drug is a measure of the percentage of the oral dose which actually reaches the systemic circulation. This can vary from the 6% bioavailability of bromocriptine to the near 100% bioavailability of glipizide. Of course, the precise bioavailability is not important as such, but it does mean that for drugs such as bromocriptine, much larger oral doses have to be given to achieve a given plasma drug level and the crucial fact is whether such large oral doses are tolerated by the stomach.

However, having reached the arterial plasma, the struggle for any drug to reach its site of action is not necessarily finished. Many drugs undergo a high degree of protein binding in plasma and only the free drug is available to exert its therapeutic effect. Glibenclamide is the perfect example of such a drug since 98%–100% is bound to plasma albumin. Changes in the degree of protein binding in patients with hypoalbuminaemia may complicate the interpretation of pharmacokinetic data but are of little direct therapeutic importance.

The above refers to the general principles involved in a drug reaching its site of action, but the other important facet of clinical pharmacology is drug elimination (or clearance). Drugs can generally be eliminated by excretion of the parent drug by the kidney or by metabolism in the liver. The former predominantly occurs with water-soluble drugs and the latter with lipid-soluble drugs. Most drugs in endocrine use are metabolised by the liver but chlorpropamide and metformin are two drugs which are eliminated by the kidney. Both drugs are therefore best avoided in renal failure.

The most important determinant of drug action is its half-life in the body, but it must be appreciated that for various reasons duration of pharmacological effect and plasma drug levels do not correspond in all cases. Often duration of effect is longer than plasma drug levels would suggest. There are two principal reasons for this. Firstly, metabolism of the parent drug may produce a metabolite which also has pharmacological activity. Indeed for some drugs such as carbimazole, the parent drug is inactive while the metabolite, methimazole, is the active ingredient. The second reason for a dissociation between plasma drug level and therapeutic effect is that the active drug becomes concentrated in some "tissue pool" within the body where it continues to exert its therapeutic effect while the drug has disappeared from the plasma. This is particularly true of glipizide, the pharmacokinetic half-life of which is about 3 hours although a significant hypoglycaemic effect is seen even after it has disappeared from the plasma.

Each group of drugs will now be considered in more detail.

Drugs Affecting Thyroid Function (see Chapter 1)

Carbimazole

Carbimazole is rapidly and completely transformed into methimazole which is the active antithyroid substance. The bioavailability of carbimazole varies greatly from one individual to another but the peak plasma concentration usually occurs 60 minutes after ingestion. The plasma half-life thereafter is quoted as 5–9 hours. Not only are there quite marked interindividual pharmacokinetic differences but, in addition, some studies suggest that methimazole elimination is enhanced in the hyperthyroid and inhibited in the hypothyroid state. Hyperthyroidism also enhances hepatic microsomal drug metabolism in general and this is most relevant in this context to β-blockers such as propranolol and metoprolol. Therefore as a hyperthyroid patient become euthyroid, propranolol and metoprolol will undergo less presystemic metabolism which increases their bioavailability.

Pharmacokinetic data do not correlate well temporally with antithyroid activity. The ability of methimazole to inhibit thyroid hormone biosynthesis involves inhibition of thyroid peroxidase and an interaction with thyroglobulin. These processes are poorly understood but methimazole appears to be accumulated within the thyroid gland in vivo. Thus the lack of a temporal correlation between plasma drug levels and antithyroid drug effects is due to the accumulation of drug in a "tissue pool" within the body. Perchlorate discharge tests suggest that despite its short kinetic half-life, methimazole inhibits iodide organification for 13 hours after a 20 mg dose. This is why carbimazole may be administered once daily rather than the t.d.s. dosage which was normal practice in the past.

It is now appreciated that part of the mechanism of action of methimazole is as an immunosuppressant. This is particularly relevant since most patients with hyperthyroidism have circulating thyroid-stimulating immunoglobulins.

One point of practical importance is that methimazole crosses the placenta, and can therefore cause hypothyroidism in the fetus. This is why the dose of carbimazole should be as low as possible in pregnancy. Methimazole is one of the few drugs to cross into breast milk to a clinically significant extent. Hence breast-feeding should be discouraged in those on carbimazole therapy.

Thyroxine

The original treatment for hypothyroidism was thyroid extract, a variable mixture of T_4 and T_3, but this has been superseded by pure synthetic thyroxine. This is despite the fact that T_4 is a relatively inactive prohormone requiring conversion to T_3 in peripheral tissues. In addition, during T_4 replacement therapy, the ratio of T_4 to T_3 is increased. Because of this, if T_4 overreplacement is suspected, this is best assessed by measurements of free T_3 rather than by measurements of plasma T_4 levels themselves.

Absorption of thyroxine is not only incomplete but is also extremely variable, especially when taken with food. For this reason thyroxine should be taken while fasting. Once absorbed, thyroxine undergoes presystemic liver metabolism and enterohepatic circulation. Hence drugs such as cholestyramine which bind bile salts inhibit the ultimate absorption of thyroxine.

Thyroxine is highly (99%) protein bound, mainly to thyroxine-binding globulin. The elimination half-life of T_4 is 6–7 days in euthyroid individuals but is increased to 9–10 days in hypothyroid patients and decreased to 3 days in hyperthyroidism. Clearly therefore, thyroxine therapy should only be given once daily.

During thyroxine replacement therapy, it is often said that the temporal relationship between the blood sample and the ingestion of thyroxine is of no consequence. Recently, however, it has been shown that plasma levels of T_4 and free T_4 are elevated for 1–6 hours after drug administration. No such changes were seen in T_3 or TSH levels, which is a further reason for using the latter measurements to judge the adequacy of T_4 replacement therapy rather than T_4 levels themselves.

Drugs Affecting Adrenocortical Function (see Chapter 2)

Glucocorticoids

The principal naturally occurring glucocorticoid is cortisol, also known as hydrocortisone. Cortisone is its inactive metabolite but it is systemically interconvertible with cortisol so that either can be administered to achieve the same pharmacological effect.

The pharmacokinetics of cortisol are complex because they are dose-dependent. This is also called non-linear kinetics since if twice the drug is administered, the plasma drug level is not twice as high. The bioavailability of cortisol varies from 45% to 80% so that as the oral dose is increased, proportionately less drug is absorbed. Cortisol is highly (90%) protein-bound, mostly to a specific high-affinity α_1 glycoprotein known as corticosteroid-binding globulin (CBG). Interestingly the amount of unbound cortisol is higher in the morning than in the afternoon, suggesting that the higher morning cortisol secretion may begin to saturate CBG and increase the free fraction.

It appears that the clearance of cortisol is also dose-related, increasing from 190 ml/min for a 5 mg dose to 500 ml/min for a 50 mg dose. Therefore it is worth noting that as the dose of cortisol is increased, less drug is absorbed and its rate of removal is increased, all of which make precise dosing of lesser importance.

The liver is a major site of steroid elimination and it is.thus relevant in two major ways. Firstly liver disease causes decreased clearance and increased half-life for cortisol. Secondly many other drugs (phenytoin, phenobarbitone, carbamazepine, rifampicin) induce microsomal oxidising enzymes in the liver and concomitant administration of these drugs can double the clearance of cortisol.

Fludrocortisone

Fludrocortisone is the commonest mineralocorticoid in clinical use. It is rapidly and completely absorbed after oral administration, reaching peak blood levels at 4–8 hours. It is 70%–80% bound to plasma proteins, especially globulins. In man, excretion occurs mainly by renal elimination (80%). In addition, a variable amount of fludrocortisone is excreted in bile, some of which is reabsorbed in the intestine and some of which is excreted in the faeces.

Fludrocortisone acts on the distal tubules of the kidneys to enhance sodium reabsorption and increases urinary potassium excretion. In larger doses it inhibits adrenocortical and ACTH secretion, promotes the deposition of liver glycogen and induces negative nitrogen balance.

Because of its potent pressor effect, it is important to adjust the dose carefully. In any individual, blood pressure, plasma electrolytes and plasma renin activity should be monitored in order to avoid over- or undertreatment.

Drugs Affecting Pituitary Function (see Chapter 5)

Bromocriptine

Dopamine agonist drugs such as bromocriptine have revolutionised the treatment of many pituitary tumours. They are of most use in prolactinomas and acromegaly but are also valuable in Parkinson's disease and in the suppression of lactation.

Bromocriptine is subject to so much incomplete absorption and first pass metabolism that only about 6% of the absorbed dose reaches the systemic circulation as parent drug. Bromocriptine is thus subject to extensive liver metabolism with the formation of a large number of different metabolites, many of which are excreted in bile. Bromocriptine, once absorbed, is extensively (90%–96%) bound to plasma protein.

There is a fairly close correlation between plasma bromocriptine levels and the suppression of prolactin levels. Peak drug levels occur about 2 hours after ingestion and disappear from plasma at about 11 hours. The suppression of prolactin and growth hormone follow a similar time profile, which is why a thrice-daily regime is standard practice to provide continuous hormonal suppression.

Drugs Affecting Calcium and Bone Metabolism (see Chapter 6)

Calcitonin

Calcitonin is used in the management of Paget's disease of bone but there are three different species of origin: human, porcine or salmon. Oddly enough salmon calcitonin is 30 times as potent as human calcitonin in altering plasma calcium and plasma cyclic AMP levels. Numerous studies have sought a pharmacokinetic explanation for these different potencies. Although absorption from the subcutaneous site is similar for each form of calcitonin, there are variations in clearance rates. Salmon calcitonin is eliminated three times as slowly as porcine calcitonin, with an intermediate value for human calcitonin. Therefore only a small part of the 30-times higher potency of salmon calcitonin can be attributed to pharmacokinetic differences. It must be concluded that the intrinsic activity of the salmon form at the receptor site is higher than that of the human or porcine forms.

After subcutaneous injection, maximum plasma concentrations of calcitonin occur 30 minutes later and disappear from the circulation within 12 hours. Salmon and human calcitonin are primarily degraded in the kidney while porcine calcitonin is mainly metabolised in the liver. Appropriate dosage adjustments must therefore be made, especially in renal impairment.

Drugs Affecting Pancreatic Function (see Chapter 7)

Insulin

Insulin is always administered parenterally because it would otherwise be destroyed by gastrointestinal enzymes. If soluble insulin were to be injected intravenously, its half-life would be about 9 minutes due to degradation in both liver and kidney.

Insulin used therapeutically is either of bovine, porcine or human origin. Bovine insulin differs from human insulin by two amino acids while porcine insulin differs by only one amino acid. Hence bovine insulin is more antigenic than porcine insulin. In the last few years, human insulin has become available. This is prepared either by chemical modification of porcine insulin or by recombinant DNA technology using *E. coli*.

In order to prolong its biological action, insulin is given by subcutaneous injection, thereby slowing its rate of delivery to the circulation. Absorption can be slowed further by combining the insulin either with protamine (a basic protein) or with zinc or with both. Isophane and lente insulins are the two main types of insulins with a prolonged duration of action. Isophane insulins are a suspension of insulin with protamine while lente insulins are a complex mixture of two types of insulin–zinc suspensions. These insulins are usually mixed within the same syringe with short-acting insulins, but it is now appreciated that zinc-containing insulins cause some delay in the onset of action of the short-acting component, while this does not occur when soluble insulins are mixed with isophane insulin.

With the recent advent of human insulins, much attention has been directed towards comparing the glycaemic and immunological profiles of human and non-human insulins. All studies agree that insulin antibody levels are reduced during therapy with human insulins. This favoured immunogenicity does reduce lipoatrophy and local allergic reactions at injection sites. With regard to glycaemic control, there are numerous data to suggest that human insulins have an accelerated absorption rate and a shorter duration of effect. This produces early hypoglycaemia and late hyperglycaemia. However there are also data to suggest that any pharmacokinetic difference between human and porcine insulins is so small that they can be used interchangeably without any change in dosage required. Therefore the prescriber should at least be aware of this potential pharmacokinetic difference. One insulin for which this appears particularly relevant is Humulin Zn, which is a crystalline insulin–zinc suspension. Although Humulin Zn is an "ultralente" type of insulin, its speed of onset and duration of action are more akin to those of a porcine "lente" insulin. It is worth noting that mean blood glucose levels are the same during treatment with human or porcine insulins and this is to be expected since early hypoglycaemia is balanced by later hyperglycaemia.

Sulphonylureas

The commonest sulphonylureas in clinical use nowadays are glibenclamide and glipizide. There are also many pharmacokinetic similarities between these two drugs.

The bioavailabilities of glibenclamide and glipizide are high, with values of 90% and 100% respectively. Peak plasma levels for both drugs occur at approximately 2 hours and their half-lives thereafter are 2–3 hours. In addition, both drugs are 98% bound to plasma protein and both are excreted by liver metabolism. The principal metabolite of glibenclamide has a weak hypoglycaemic effect but this is of little clinical significance at therapeutic doses.

Another similarity between the two drugs is that their hypoglycaemic effect persists even after plasma drug levels have disappeared. The precise reason for this is poorly understood but it is not due to active metabolites. When glipizide is given as a single morning dose, it still exerts a hypoglycaemic effect in the evening and through until the next morning. However, in one of the few comparisons between different drug regimens, it was found that evening blood glucose control was better when glibenclamide was given as two divided doses rather than as a single morning dose. Thus blood glucose control is often adequate on once-daily dosing but may be improved by dividing drug doses. Their main adverse effect is hypoglycaemia but skin rashes, cholestatic jaundice and gastrointestinal symptoms can occur.

Less commonly used nowadays are chlorpropamide and tolbutamide. Chlorpropamide is a unique sulphonylurea in several ways. It is excreted by the kidney while all others are metabolised by the liver. In addition, the ingestion of alcohol can cause skin flushing in about one-third of all patients taking chlorpropamide. High-dose aspirin can decrease renal excretion and therefore potentiate the effect of chlorpropamide. Finally, chlorpropamide has more of an antidiuretic effect than other sulphonylureas and should therefore be avoided in cardiac and renal failure.

Tolbutamide is a highly protein-bound drug with a short duration of action. This latter effect makes it most suitable for elderly patients. It is, however, worth noting that both phenylbutazone and warfarin will increase the hypoglycaemic effect of tolbutamide especially. This is due both to inhibition of liver metabolism and to displacement of drug from protein-binding sites.

Metformin

The clinical pharmacology of metformin has attracted much attention and research. This is due to an obvious desire to identify the risk factors which encourage the development of biguanide-induced lactic acidosis. This serious though uncommon problem is commoner in the presence of cardiac, renal or hepatic dysfunction, all of which are now considered contraindications to metformin. Much commoner as side-effects of metformin in routine practice are nausea, vomiting and diarrhoea.

Metformin has been found to behave pharmacokinetically in a rather curious manner, described as "flip-flop" kinetics. This is because, unusually, the rate of absorption is slower than the rate of elimination. Therefore the decline in plasma drug level is governed by the rate of absorption rather than the rate of elimination. This is due mainly to its slow gastrointestinal absorption although in addition its elimination from plasma is rapid, with a half-life of 1.5 hours after intravenous dosing. Its brief half-life makes it unlikely that significant drug accumulation would occur during chronic therapy. This may explain the lower incidence of toxic effects such as lactic acidosis than after phenformin.

Oral bioavailability is 50%–60% with some drug becoming bound to the intestinal wall. None of the drug is protein-bound in plasma. Metformin is eliminated by active secretion through the kidney and its half-life is extended to 5 hours in the presence of renal impairment.

Metformin is thought to act by reducing hepatic glucose production. It is generally administered twice or thrice daily. Pharmacological effect correlates temporally with plasma drug levels. Gastrointestinal absorption is so slow that effective plasma drug levels are present for 8–12 hours after drug ingestion.

Further Reading

General

Hall R, Anderson J, Smart GA, Besser M (eds) (1980) Fundamentals of clinical endocrinology, 3rd edn. Pitman Medical, Tunbridge Wells
Williams RH (ed) (1985) Textbook of endocrinology, 7th edn. Saunders, Philadelphia

Thyroid

Oppenheimer JH (ed) (1977) Thyroid today (series). Travenol Laboratories, Deerfield, Illinois
Werner SC, Ingbar SH (eds) (1986) The thyroid, 5th edn. Harper & Row, Hagerstown, Maryland

Adrenal

Anderson DC, Winter JDS (eds) (1985) Clinical endocrinology: adrenal cortex. Butterworth, London
James VHT (ed) (1979) Comprehensive endocrinology: the adrenal gland. Raven Press, New York

Pituitary

Beardwell L, Robertson GL (1981) Clinical endocrinology, vol 1, The pituitary. Butterworth, London
Belchetz P (ed) (1984) Management of pituitary disease. Chapman & Hall, London
Laws ER Jr, Randall RV, Kern EB, Abboud CF (eds) (1982) Management of pituitary adenomas and related lesions with emphasis on transsphenoidal microsurgery. Appleton-Century-Crofts, New York

Calcium and Bone

Heath DA, Marx SJ (1982) Clinical endocrinology, vol 2, Calcium disorders. Butterworth, London
Nordin BEC (ed) (1984) Metabolic bone and stone disease. Churchill Livingstone, Edinburgh

Pancreas

Johnston D (ed) (1982) New aspects of diabetes. Clin Endocrinol Metab 11(2)
Keen H, Jarrett J (eds) (1982) Complications of diabetes, 2nd edn Edward Arnold, London
Marks V, Rose FC (eds) (1981) Hypoglycaemia, 2nd edn. Blackwell Scientific, Oxford
National Diabetes Data Group (1985) Diabetes in America. NIH publication 85-1468. US Department of Health and Human Services
Schade DS (ed) (1983) Metabolic acidosis. Clin Endocrinol Metab 12(2)
Watkins PJ (1983) ABC of diabetes. British Medical Association, London

Pharmacopoeia

1. The Thyroid Gland

Hypothyroidism

L-thyroxine is usually prescribed at a starting dose of 50 µg once daily by mouth, increasing the dose by 50 µg at 2-weekly intervals until full replacement (100–200 µg daily) is achieved. Full replacement is assessed by biochemical results after 3 months of treatment. The drug is given once daily as it has a half-life of 7 days. Care must be taken instituting replacement in those patients with ischaemic heart disease.

Triiodothyronine is usually prescribed at a starting dose of 2.5–5 µg 8-hourly, increasing gradually to 10 µg 8-hourly over a period of 1 week. If the patient is stable on this dose, treatment with L-thyroxine can be commenced at a dose of 100 µg once daily and the oral triiodothyronine withdrawn after a 3-day overlap.

Hyperthyroidism

Carbimazole interferes with thyroid hormone synthesis and may act as an immunosuppressant. It is converted in the body to its active metabolite methimazole. Despite having a short plasma half-life the prolonged biological effect of carbimazole permits a once-daily administration. Doses of 20 mg once daily are usually adequate to control thyroid function, but the effect of the drug should be titrated by its clinical effect coupled with serial estimation of plasma thyroid hormones. Patients should be treated with carbimazole for a minimum of 6 months to a maximum of 1 year; the remission rate following withdrawal is somewhere in the region of 30% in patients with Graves' disease. Patients should be warned of the risk of skin rash and agranulocytosis.

Propylthiouracil is more protein-bound than methimazole and is given in doses 10 times that of carbimazole. It is more suitable than carbimazole for breast-feeding mothers as less of the drug is secreted in breast milk. Although the biological half-life of propylthiouracil is less than that of carbimazole it can be given as a once-daily dose.

Potassium iodide when given in a dose of 60 mg 8-hourly will reduce thyroid hormone levels to normal in the majority of patients by the tenth day of treatment, but prolonged treatment with this drug cannot be recommended as thyroid hormones may rise again after this period. It is therefore used as part of the preparation of a patient for thyroid surgery.

Propranolol LA is a useful drug for controlling some of the cardiovascular effects of hyperthyroidism and is given as a once-only dose of 160 mg.

Sodium ^{131}I (radioiodine) is a radiopharmaceutical that is usually prescribed under the auspices of a nuclear medicine department. In Graves' disease a single dose of 10 mc (370 MBq) ^{131}I will achieve remission in 88% of patients at 1 year, with hypothyroidism in 61% at 1 year; the subsequent hypothyroid rate is approximately 3.4% per annum. In uninodular goitre a single dose of 15 mc (555 MBq) ^{131}I will achieve remission in 100% at 1 year with hypothyroidism in 40%. In multinodular goitre a single dose of 30 mc (740 MBq) ^{131}I will achieve remission in 74% at 1 year with hypothyroidism in 24%.

2. The Adrenal Gland: Adrenal Cortex

Hypoadrenalism

Cortisol (Hydrocortisone) is usually prescribed in a dose of 20 mg by mouth before breakfast (food delays absorption) and again in a dose of 10 mg 8 hours later. The dose should be titrated by the patient's weight, blood pressure and biochemistry. Patients should be advised to double the dose of glucocorticoid in times of acute stress such as a febrile illness or accident. They should also be encouraged to carry identification that they are on corticosteroid replacement. The relative potencies and equivalent doses of corticosteroids are as follows:

Compound	Relative anti-inflammatory potency	Relative sodium-retaining potency	Duration of action[a] (h)	Approximate equivalent dose (mg)
Cortisol	1	1	8–12	20
Prednisolone	4	0.8	12–36	5
Dexamethasone	25	0	36–72	0.75
Fludrocortisone	10	125	8–12	–

[a]Biological half-life

Fludrocortisone is employed for mineralocorticoid replacement by the oral administration of a once-daily dose of 0.05–0.3 mg. The dose is titrated by measurement of blood pressure, plasma electrolytes and plasma renin activity.

Hyperadrenalism

Metyrapone may be given in a dose of 250 mg 6-hourly to prepare patients with Cushing's syndrome for surgery; the dose is titrated to the plasma coritsol profile throughout the day to maintain plasma cortisol levels between 330 and 400 nmol/l.

o,p'-**DDD** is a compound related to the insecticide DDT. It has a relatively selective cytotoxic action upon adenocortical cells and is therefore used in the treatment of undetectable adrenocortical tumours. The drug is administered by mouth in three divided doses of 5–15 g daily. After discontinuation of therapy the drug is still present in plasma for up to 3 months. The dose of the drug should be titrated to the plasma cortisol profile throughout the day. Side- effects include anorexia and nausea (80%), lethargy (35%) and dermatitis (20%), and the dose of the drug may have to be reduced.

Dexamethasone given in a dose of 0.5–1 mg last thing before retiring will usually suppress the hypothalamic–pituitary–adrenal axis in children with congenital adrenal hyperplasia and reduce adrenal androgen secretion. Care must be taken in adjusting the dose to suppress adrenal androgen secretion sufficiently without giving excessive glucocorticoid. Androgen excess will result in premature fusion of the epiphyses whilst glucocorticoid excess will inhibit growth.

The Adrenal Gland: Adrenal Medulla

Phaeochromocytoma

Phenoxybenzamine is a non-competitive α-adrenergic receptor antagonist with prolonged effect. Treatment is begun with doses of 20–40 mg daily and increased if necessary until adequate blood pressure control is achieved. α-Adrenoceptor blockade should be introduced before β-adrenoceptor blockade otherwise elevation rather than reduction of blood pressure may occur.

Propranolol is administered orally in doses of 40–80 mg 8-hourly to achieve β-adrenoceptor blockade and prevent cardiac arrhythmias.

Sodium nitroprusside is a peripheral arterio- and veno-dilator with a rapid onset of action of 1–2 minutes and rapid dissipation on stopping the infusion. Used with care it is an excellent drug for controlling intra-operative changes in blood pressure that occur with handling of phaeochromocytomas. Nitroprusside 50 mg is dissolved in 500 ml of 5% glucose producing a concentration of 100 µg/ml. The usual rate of infusion is 0.5–10 µg/kg/min and the dose is titrated to blood pressure levels. Only fresh solutions should be used and the bottle should be covered with an opaque wrapping as the compound decomposes in light.

3. The Ovary

Hypogonadism

Ethinyloestradiol 10–20 µg once daily by mouth from days 1 to 21 of the menstrual cycle and **medroxyprogesterone acetate** 5 mg once daily by mouth from days 14 to 21 of the cycle is a useful combination for sex steroid replacement therapy. Withdrawal of sex steroids from days 22 to 28 results in menstruation, and cyclical treatment is restarted on day 1.

Clomiphene is an anti-oestrogen preparation preventing the normal "feed-back inhibition" control of oestrogen synthesis by the hypothalamus and pituitary resulting in increased secretion of GnRH and gonadotrophins. An oral dose of 50–100 mg once daily is given on days 1 to 5 of each menstrual cycle and the response may be monitored by estimation of the day 21 plasma progesterone concentration. It is used for induction of ovulation and to restore normal menstrual cycles. Side-effects include disturbance of peripheral vision, particularly at dawn and dusk.

Gonadotrophin therapy is used to induce ovulation and fertility in those patients with secondary gonadal failure, for whom clomiphene is ineffective. Treatment involves two stages. Menotrophin (human menopausal gonadotrophin) is administered daily in a dose of 75–150 units by intramuscular injection until follicular development is adequate. The response must be carefully monitored with ovarian ultrasound and estimation of plasma oestrogen concentrations. When plasma oestrogen concentrations of between 1100 and 3000 pmol/l have been achieved a single intramuscular dose of hCG (10 000 units) is given to induce ovulation. The complications of this form of treatment include hyperstimulation syndrome and multiple pregnancy.

GnRH therapy is delivered to patients with secondary gonadal failure by means of a portable pulsatile pump (Graesby) that mimics the natural secretion of GnRH. A dose of 10–20 µg is given subcutaneously every 90 minutes and treatment should be continued until a pregnancy is achieved or for a maximum period of 6 months.

Hypergonadism

GnRH analogues are synthetic analogues of naturally occurring GnRH differing by an amino acid substitution that increases their potency and prolongs their biological half-life. Their administration causes "down-regulation" of anterior pituitary GnRH receptors resulting in a hypogonado-trophic hypogonadism. These agents are therefore potentially useful in controlling precocious puberty. Buserelin (Hoechst) may be given by the intranasal route in doses of 200 µg twice daily; Zoladex (ICI) may be given as depot preparation in a dose of 3.6 mg by intramuscular injection once monthly but is not yet widely available.

Dexamethasone given by mouth in doses of 0.5–1 mg last thing before retiring can successfully reduce plasma testosterone levels in hirsute women. It acts by suppressing both the adrenal gland and the ovary. However, an impaired cortisol response to stress is an undesirable consequence. This regimen may also be used to control excessive adrenal androgen secretion in children with congenital adrenal hyperplasia.

Cyproterone Acetate is an anti-androgen acting as a competitive antagonist of testosterone and is used in the treatment of hirsutism. Since this drug has progestogen-like activity and has a prolonged half-life it is usually given with oestrogen in a reversed sequential regimen. This regimen is also contracep-tive, preventing the possible exposure of a male fetus to an anti-androgen in utero. Ethinyloestradiol 50 µg daily is administered by mouth from days 5 to 21 of the menstrual cycle and cyproterone acetate 100 mg daily from days 5 to 15 of the cycle. The treatment is continued cyclically, with a withdrawal bleed between days 21 and 28.

Spironolactone is also a competitive antagonist of testosterone as well as being an inhibitor of 5α-reductase, and is employed in the treatment of hirsutism. The drug is administered in a dose of 50–75 mg once daily by mouth and has few side-effects. However, abnormal uterine bleeding may occur in mid-cycle and if this becomes a problem it should be treated by the addition of an oral contraceptive agent.

4. The Testis

Hypogonadism

Testosterone replacement therapy can usually be achieved either by the oral administration of testosterone undecanoate 40–80 mg 12-hourly, the intra-muscular injection of testosterone esters (Sustanon 250) 1 ampoule every 3–4 weeks, or by the subcutaneous implantation of testosterone pellets (600 mg) every 6 months.

Gonadotrophin therapy involves the stimulation of testosterone secretion from the Leydig cells in patients with secondary gonadal failure by the intramuscular administration of hCG 1500 units twice weekly. Spermatogenesis is induced by the concomitant intramuscular administration of menotropin 150 units three times weekly. Treatment is for a minimum period of 6 months.

GnRH therapy is delivered to patients with secondary gonadal failure by means of a pulsatile pump (Graesby) in a dose of approximately 5 μg subcutaneously every 90 minutes. The response should be monitored by estimation of plasma testosterone levels, semen analysis and plasma gonadotrophins. Treatment should be continued for a minimum of 6 months.

Hypergonadism

GnRH analogues in the treatment of precocious puberty has been discussed under the section "The Ovary".

5. The Pituitary Gland

Hypopituitarism

Replacement of cortisol, thyroxine and steroids is discussed under the appropriate sections. Patients with secondary adrenal failure do not require mineralocorticoid replacement therapy as may those with primary adrenal failure. Care must be taken in treating hypopituitarism with thyroxine replacement alone as this may precipitate adrenocortical failure in patients with concomitant glucocorticoid insufficiency. Cortisol and thyroxine replacement should be administered concomitantly in these patients.

Growth hormone is currently synthesised by recombinant DNA technology and is administered by intramuscular injection 10 units twice weekly for children with growth failure. If growth failure is associated with panhypopituitarism care must be taken in balancing the replacement of glucocorticoid and sex steroids so as not to cause premature fusion of the epiphyses.

Desmopressin is a long-acting synthetic vasopressin analogue with little pressor activity, employed for the treatment of cranial diabetes insipidus. Usually 10–20 μg is given by the nasal route once or twice daily using a rhinyle, or 1–2 μg by the intramuscular route. Plasma electrolytes should be estimated to monitor therapy.

Pituitary Tumours

Bromocriptine is a dopamine agonist which is employed in inhibiting prolactin secretion by prolactin-secreting pituitary tumours and shrinking the size of macroprolactinomas even if there has been extension above the sella compressing the visual pathways. Treatment with this drug is an alternative to neurosurgery and can be considered as first-line therapy, followed by external pituitary irradiation for larger tumours. Bromocriptine cannot be considered as first-line treatment for hGH-secreting tumours as this drug usually only achieves a 50% reduction of plasma hGH concentrations, but it is a useful adjunct where plasma hGH remains elevated following surgery and whilst radiotherapy is taking effect.

Bromocriptine is introduced cautiously in a dose of 1.25 mg orally with a snack on going to bed, as it may cause postural hypotension, nausea and vomiting. On waking the next day the patient can take a further 1.25 mg if there were no adverse side-effects. The dose can be gradually increased by 1.25 mg daily increments to 2.5 mg 8-hourly for the treatment of prolactinomas and 5–10 mg 8-hourly for the treatment of hGH-secreting tumours.

6. Calcium and Bones

Hypocalcaemia

Effervescent calcium (Sandocal) contains 5.23 g calcium lactate-gluconate and 0.8 g calcium carbonate equivalent to 1 g of elemental calcium. One tablet daily is usually sufficient in cases of osteomalacia, osteoporosis and hypocalcaemia.

Intravenous calcium gluconate is indicated in cases of severe hypocalcaemia. Initially 10 ml 10% calcium gluconate is given followed by an infusion of 1.7 ml/kg in either saline or glucose 5% over a 4-hour period. Concomitant magnesium deficiency should also be corrected.

Alphacalcidol is the 1α-OH metabolite of vitamin D_3 and has a more rapid course of action than vitamin D_3 itself. It is prescribed in "high" doses of 1–3 μg daily by mouth for cases of vitamin D deficiency, osteomalacia, rickets, malabsorption and renal failure. It should not be used to treat patients with environmental osteomalacia (see text for details) as this may respond to a course of ultraviolet irradiation or "low-dose" vitamin D_3 therapy (calcium with vitamin D tablets containing 12.5 μg calciferol and 2 mmol calcium).

Osteoporosis

Ethinyloestradiol treatment for osteoporosis is discussed under the section "The Ovary".

Paget's Disease

Salmon calcitonin is a synthetic calcitonin used in the treatment of Paget's disease of the bone and hypercalcaemia. In Paget's disease 100 units daily is given by subcutaneous injection, reducing to 50–100 units three times weekly after 1 month; treatment is usually continued for 1 year. Therapy should be monitored by estimation of plasma calcium concentrations, plasma alkaline phosphatase and urinary hydroxyproline excretion. Side-effects include flushing of the face and hands, diarrhoea and vomiting and a skin rash. Higher doses of 400 units 8-hourly are used for the treatment of hypercalcaemia.

Disodium Etidronate is an oral agent used in the treatment of symptomatic Paget's disease. A single dose (initially 5 mg/kg) is given once daily 2 hours before food for a period not exceeding 6 months. Side-effects include gastrointestinal disturbance and the development of focal osteomalacia, so prolonged use of the drug cannot be recommended. However, treatment can be given cyclically (see text for details).

7. The Endocrine Pancreas

Hyperglycaemia

Metformin is a biguanide inhibiting hepatic glucose production used as an oral hypoglycaemic agent in the treatment of obese diabetics in conjunction with a weight-reducing diet. It has several unpleasant side-effects including anorexia, malaise, vomiting and diarrhoea and it is these properties that probably permit weight loss despite improved blood glucose control. Lactic acidosis is a potential and more serious side-effect and metformin should not be prescribed in patients with either liver disease or renal impairment. (The drug is excreted by the kidney.) Doses should not exceed 850 mg 12-hourly.

Chlorpropamide is a long-acting sulphonylurea with a biological half-life of 36 hours used for the treatment of non-obese diabetics in conjunction with a diabetic diet. It acts by stimulating insulin secretion in response to glucose and enhancing insulin action. Side-effects include skin rash, jaundice, agranulocytosis and facial flushing in response to alcohol. It is administered by mouth in doses of 100–375 mg once daily. Glipizide is an alternative drug with a much shorter half-life of approximately 5 hours. It is therefore more suitable for elderly patients, in whom hypoglycaemia may be a serious complication of chlorpropamide therapy.

Insulins may be classified according to their source, purity and duration of action. However, the recent developments in the manufacture of insulin have enabled the production of highly purified human insulin either by enzymatic manipulation of porcine insulin (semi-synthetic) or by recombinant DNA technology. Clearly human insulin will be the source of future insulin production. Insulins are therefore divided according to the speed of onset and the duration of their action:

Short-acting insulins (Actrapid, Novo) are unmodified and have a plasma half-life of 5 minutes and a biological half-life of approximately 20 minutes when given intravenously. Intramuscular injection prolongs the half-life to up to 2 hours and the subcutaneous route is employed for maintenance therapy. The time to onset of action is approximately 30 minutes, and the duration of action 6 hours. However, variations in injection technique can alter this considerably.

Medium-acting insulins (Monotard, Novo) are modified as an insulin–zinc suspension (30% amorphous and 70% crystalline). The time to onset of action is 1–3 hours and the duration of action 7–15 hours.

Long-acting insulins (Ultratard, Novo) are also modified as an insulin–zinc suspension (crystalline). Their time to onset of action is 3 hours and duration of action 10–24 hours.

Various regimens employing a combination of insulins to maintain adequate blood sugar control are illustrated in the text.

Hypoglycaemia

Glucagon should be issued to every insulin-treated diabetic for use in combating serious hypoglycaemia. The dose is 1 mg given by intramuscular injection. It is often wise to educate the patient's family in the emergency administration of this drug.

Subject Index